Decolonising Public Health through Praxis

Faye Bruce • Ornette D. Clennon

Decolonising Public Health through Praxis

The Impact on Black Health in the UK

palgrave
macmillan

Faye Bruce
Department of Nursing, Brooks Building
Manchester Metropolitan University
Manchester, UK

Ornette D. Clennon
MaCTRI, Brow House
MEaP
Manchester, UK

ISBN 978-3-031-18407-9   ISBN 978-3-031-18405-5   (eBook)
https://doi.org/10.1007/978-3-031-18405-5

Cover pattern © Melisa Hasan

This Palgrave Macmillan imprint is published by the registered company Springer Nature Switzerland AG.
The registered company address is: Gewerbestrasse 11, 6330 Cham, Switzerland

Preface

I am very pleased and honoured that this volume marks the first contribution to the book series, *Palgrave Studies in Decolonisation and Grassroots Black Organic Intellectualism*. In these current troubled times, we desperately need clear thinking and mature praxis around how decolonisation can be made useful in liberating and empowering grassroots communities. As will be explored by future contributions to the series, the rise of populism and ethno-nationalism are forcing grassroots communities around the world to fight for their very existence, as they confront their increasingly unstable nation states. Although not as openly visceral, grassroots communities in the UK are also fighting equally hard for their existence, a fight that involves protecting their civil (human) rights to local services. Nowhere is this felt more keenly than in the field of health. In the UK, the instability of the state is represented by a diminishing National Health Service (NHS) and an equally diminishing priority of an equitable healthcare system that works for everyone. This volume and the wider book series aim to make visible the not-so-hidden reasons why inequity is felt more keenly by some more than by others.

The scholarship in this volume and across the series is intended to both illuminate and agitate questions at both grassroots and policy levels to ask what can be done to make positive changes and what are the mindsets that stubbornly prevent positive change from taking place.

It is urgent that grassroots communities and policy makers grasp the ethical and moral nettle of inequitable healthcare because the health of the *entire* nation depends on it.

Manchester, UK   Ornette D. Clennon

Acknowledgements

We would like to thank God without whom none of this would have happened. We would also like to thank all of our community partners, whose voices in this volume form a golden thread of community wisdom whose absence would have made the writing of this volume impossible.

Ornette D. Clennon

I would like to thank my colleagues and work family at MEaP (Making Education a Priority: Dr Esther Oludipe, Jumoke Quadri, Amber Abisai, Henry Ngawoofah and Christina Ntow), who supported me in co-writing this book. I would also like to especially thank Professor T. J. Curry for his insightful suggestions that helped to broaden our scholarly enquiry. Lastly but not least, I would like to thank my co-author for her golden community insights.

Faye Bruce

It has been a pleasure working alongside my co-author, who has been instrumental in the creative design and many scholarly aspects of this book. I am so grateful to the Chief Executive Charles Kwaku-Odoi of the Caribbean & African Health Network, who has been highly strategic and operational in the development of the organisation which is the bedrock of what we do to support and enable our communities. Finally, I would like to thank the Black communities for giving us the mandate to advocate for them to tackle the health and well-being concerns in our communities and hence help to meet our vision to reduce health inequalities for Black people in a generation.

Contents

1

Introduction: How Does the African Diaspora Health-Seeker Fair in the Current Health Market in the UK?

Abstract In this chapter, we will introduce our decolonial reading of whiteness as a lens through which to present the current landscape of Public Health for African Diaspora communities in the UK. The chapter will also identify the *hidden factors* for systemic failure for the African Diaspora health seeker and locate them within a "coloniality of whiteness". To do this, we will introduce whiteness as an unethical framework (i.e. a distortion of Aristotelian human ethics) for social ordering that can be traced back to *historical patterns of behaviour* over the longue durée. We will also introduce the notion of the "grassroots Black organic intellectual" as being the conduit for such decolonial analyses of whiteness in the community, which will form a decolonial praxis that will be threaded throughout the volume.

Keywords Human ethics • Whiteness • Decoloniality • Decolonisation • Communities

© The Author(s), under exclusive license to Springer Nature Switzerland AG 2022   1
F. Bruce, O. D. Clennon, *Decolonising Public Health through Praxis*,
https://doi.org/10.1007/978-3-031-18405-5_1

Introduction

The Health Landscape for African Diaspora (Black) Health Seekers

In the UK health system, it is recognised that the health experiences of Black people are poorer due to unequal access to health services and a lack of appropriate care in comparison to those from white majority communities (populations). For instance, there is much evidence that identifies how difficult late-stage diagnoses are to treat across a number of conditions (e.g. Berwald et al., 2016). To illustrate this, even though Black women are less likely to be diagnosed with breast cancer in England, they are more likely to be diagnosed with late-stage breast cancer and die as a result (BreastCancer.org, 2022). In Chap. 3, we share our own stories whilst growing up in the UK, of family friends who died at an early age because they were not listened to in their GP/patient encounter. This, of course, has resulted in a lack of trust and engagement with health practitioners, that we will explore in Chap. 4.

Healthcare is highly valued in society and the aim is to produce improved health as an outcome (Wellings, 2017). In Greater Manchester (GM), devolution has enabled a delegated transfer of power and resources from National to Local government, which covers political, fiscal and administrative responsibilities (MacKinnon, 2015). The ultimate aim of devolution in GM is to enable freedom and flexibilities from national decision-making so that they can improve health outcomes and reduce health inequalities locally (Walshe et al., 2016). Since Devolution in 2016, Black communities have not been beneficiaries of improved health inequalities from the £6 billion awarded to GM to be spent in Health and Social care. To date, Black people in GM still experience high rates of inequalities, some of which include high deaths linked to pregnancy, high rates of heart-related diseases, such as heart failure, kidney disease, stroke, diabetes, prostate cancer, mental health, HIV (GMCA, 2015) and more recently COVID-19. Nationally, the prevalence of obesity is highest among women and children of Black African descent and this is replicated within Manchester (Riches, 2016). However, there are limited targeted interventions to address this prevalence, which is a factor for cardiovascular disease (CVD).

Racism as a Social Determinant of Health

Our community partners tell us clearly that the quality of care and access varies according to race, as part of those wider social determinants impedes the ability of Black people to access the full range of health gains that is afforded to majority populations. Our partners also explain how they feel excluded from health prevention information and interventions that are not targeted towards their communities despite their risks of poor health. They speak about racial stereotypes that suggest that Black people are unlikely to comply with health initiatives. However, the healthcare system that is made up of *people*, (who write policies and direct practice) has not responded to address the lack of trust Black people have, as a result of their own and others' past experiences. Our community partners speak about how Black people have not benefited from merit goods or services such as the NHS that should deliver positive externalities for everyone. However, the merit goods that exist, do not do enough to equally and equitably meet the direct needs of Black communities, even though healthcare is provided free at the point of use. Historically, healthcare prevention has focused on a medical model to address health and illness, which resulted in the lack of attention being paid to those factors outside of biology/genetic and cultural reasons (Mantovani et al., 2017; Pinto et al., 2008).

Social determinants are a significant factor in an individual's health and can impact far greater than the amount of healthcare the individual receives from services. In comparison to white people, Black people have unequal access to well-paid employment and are more likely to be unemployed (Demie, 2021). Black people (particularly those of Caribbean origin) are more likely to have a worse education experience and disproportionately face more school exclusions (Gov.uk, 2019). Black people are less likely to live in environmentally safe conditions and tend to live in overcrowded houses (Verhaeghe & Ghekiere, 2021). So, there is actually a lot of evidence about ethnic health inequalities and their contributory factors, yet the attention in this area in terms of policy seems to have been neglected.

As will be identified throughout this volume, Black people are more likely to be subjected to racism on the basis of their physical characteristics and hence are more likely to suffer chronic health conditions including experiencing poor mental health, such as depression and anxiety. This is particularly problematic for Black people who have mental health problems because they are likely to suffer the effects of discrimination both on the basis of their race *and* on the basis of their condition. Discrimination can lead to poverty and social isolation, in addition, it can negatively impact how individuals seek healthcare. In order to identify, anticipate and prevent adverse outcomes, it is important for health service providers to understand racism and its biases as *ethical* issues that need to be redressed.

The roles that race and racism play in health inequalities have largely been ignored by public health and were not identified as a social determinant of health until the recent *Marmot Review 10 years on* (Marmot, 2020),[1] despite there being a mountain of literature that argues that cultural factors, poverty/class and or/biology are the driving forces behind health inequalities (e.g. Nazroo et al., 2009; Braveman et al., 2015; Wallace et al., 2016, etc.). More recently, Fenton et al. (2020) were tasked to carry out a government inquiry into the possible impact of ethnicity and race on COVID-19 outcomes, with a view towards bringing about a shift in policy on the health inequalities agenda. However, although their study described the differences between groups, their findings failed to analyse the *hidden factors* or the underlying the reasons.

The NHS has a poor history of care given to Caribbean and African people and studies have shown low satisfaction rates that are a measure of quality (Pinder et al., 2016; Rabiee & Smith, 2014). As will be articulated in Chap. 4, our community partners express that there is a crucial lack of targeted health prevention information in written and verbal form to empower them to be self-caring and self-managing of their own health as outlined in the NHS long-term plan (NHS, 2022). In the UK, the responsibility of health improvement is placed on individuals to make healthcare decisions that can keep them well. However, to do this, healthcare information should be accessible, universally proportionate (Marmot,

---

[1] See Chap. 5 for the role grassroots advocacy had in highlighting this issue to Sir Michael Marmot.

2010) and provide care and information that is inclusive to meet health and wellbeing needs. Yet, despite a free NHS developed on the principle of equity there are significant inequitable and unjust experiences in access to appropriate care for the Caribbean and African community (Wilson et al., 2012). There seems to be a *systematic* failure in the market to provide equitable and fair access to the healthcare benefits of the market that are stated to bring, as outlined in the NHS Constitution in England, Principle 1 of the NHS constitution:

> The NHS provides a comprehensive service, available to all. It is available to all irrespective of gender, race, disability, age, sexual orientation, religion, belief, gender reassignment, pregnancy and maternity or marital or civil partnership status. The service is designed to improve, prevent, diagnose and treat both physical and mental health problems with equal regard. It has a duty to each and every individual that it serves and must respect their human rights. At the same time, it has a wider social duty to promote equality through the services it provides and to pay particular attention to groups or sections of society where improvements in health and life expectancy are not keeping pace with the rest of the population. (Gov.uk, 2021, para 6)

Although there has been some movement towards more inclusive healthcare practices, [2] the legacy of race continues to limit Black people's access to services that can improve their health. Discrimination and bias towards racial inferiority have left Black people with lower levels of human capital and also left them unable to navigate the health service and utilise what our community partners describe as access to resources that would improve their health.

The Role of Whiteness in the Health Market

Through our many community conversations, we have identified that race and its biases are real *ethical* issues that remain *hidden factors* within the *systemic failure* of the health market to provide equal access to health

---

[2] See Chap. 5.

for African Diaspora health seekers. As a result of that, this volume will make extensive use of the voices of our community partners, as well as our own experiences. This is an important facet of the volume because as its authors, we are also embedded scholar-activists within our communities and as such, occupy the position of "grassroots Black organic intellectuals" (Gordon, 2009). Our function as organic intellectuals (cf. Gordon, 2009; Gramsci, 1999) is very much to create and hold spaces where liberatory praxis can be developed and sustained by the whole community. In practice, what this looks like, is having conversations with our community partners, as part of our community activism that fuses together theory (e.g. interdisciplinary critical race studies) with working strategies for community health-uplift and empowerment. You will read more about this in Chaps. 4 and 5.

So, for us, all of these hidden factors behind the previously mentioned systemic failures are underpinned by an ethical and moral framework of whiteness, which comprises specific *historical patterns of behaviour* that in turn, strongly underpin Eurocentric theory and praxis. This volume will attempt to trace these historical patterns of behaviour over the longue durée, as a way of establishing a foundation for a shorthand reference to whiteness that can be readily understood in wider public discourse (Clennon, 2019). In essence, we will be decolonising whiteness. Our odyssey of decolonising whiteness will embody both decolonisation as uncovering traditional pre-colonial knowledges (epistemologies) (Mignolo, 2002) of whiteness, as well as decoloniality (Mignolo, 2000), where we will uncover the remnants of colonialism (whiteness) in our modern day thinking around healthcare.

In Chap. 2, we will start by positioning whiteness as a theoretical framework that distorts Aristotle's (1944) "natural law" in his *Politics*. For us, whiteness' historical patterns of behaviour follow an unerring desire to dehumanise human beings in order to justify conquest. We strongly believe that this act of dehumanisation is both unethical and morally degenerate, in equal measure. In this chapter, we will show how this unethical and morally degenerate behaviour contradicts the human ethics of Aristotle (and the rest of the Ancient World), who firmly believed in "mankind as a whole" ([1254b] [1] lines 11–13), amongst which, his "natural slaves" and "natural rulers" were included with *equal* importance.

We will also show how this unethical distortion of Aristotelian human ethics developed into the *conception* of whiteness, when it learned to homogenise and essentialise its enemies ("others") during the Holy Crusades but as you will also see, this "favour" was *not* returned by the Mediaeval Arabic World.

We will then characterise the Valladolid debates and the emergence of "raza" (bloodlines) as the *gestation* period of whiteness, where important tools (methods) emerged to further dehumanise "others". Firstly, illustrated by a moral blindness of not seeing people for who they really were but instead seeing them through the lens of an unacknowledged (disavowed) immorality (i.e. transferring or superimposing the viewer's immorality onto the object of its gaze), which we dub the "Sepúlveda complex". And secondly, with the important embryonic notion of race ("raza") that applied ideas around animal pedigree to human beings to distinguish them for persecution (ethnic cleansing). We then see the *birth* of whiteness, in the invention of "The Negro", where finally all of these tools of dehumanisation that had been developed over the centuries, coalesced and were vigorously applied to the enslaved African for the sole purpose of justifying the making of profit from its dehumanised body and labour. Using the voices of our community partners, we then will apply this ethical and moral framework of whiteness to examine the role of gatekeeping in today's health market with its deleterious effects on the African Diaspora health seeker.

In Chap. 3, we will take a closer look at "The Negro" by tracing the creation of its "gender", as shaped by imperial whiteness, during this era. We will do this primarily through a conversation between the authors about their experiences growing up in the UK; conversations that will act as gateways into exploring the echoes of past imperial structures that still have an impact on us, today (i.e. "coloniality of power" or as we call it, "coloniality of whiteness"). In this chapter, we assert that understanding the role of gender formation in Empire and how it shaped Black women and Black men in terms of the enduring stereotypes it created for them is important for understanding the prevailing and current attitudes of the healthcare sector to its African Diaspora health seekers. This will allow us to uncover more of the hidden factors behind the widespread systemic failure of the health market for the former. Related to this, we will also critique intersectionality as a serious framework for understanding health inequalities for *both* Black women and Black men.

In Chap. 4, using the voices of our community partners, we will take a deeper look into the "traditional heritage knowledges" (Clennon, 2022) around health, found in our communities. The approach we take here will be much more informed by the process of decolonisation, since, we will be using Ubuntu's (see Waghid & Smeyers, 2012) ethno-philosophical framework (Emeagwali, 2014; Sefa Dei, 2014) to excavate pre-colonial (traditional) African knowledges of health that still exist within our contemporary African Diaspora communities. And then by using Ubuntu's critical philosophy framework (Dzobo, 1992; Gyekye, 1995), we will attempt to visualise what those traditional African knowledges and their application might look like in the twenty-first century of collaboration between grassroots communities and statutory health providers.

Finally, in Chap. 5, we will present a case study of a community Black-led health advocacy organisation called Caribbean and African Health Network (CAHN), whose role is that of "grassroots Black organic intellectuals" in their communities. We will show how the knowledge of whiteness over the longue durée is being used to help African Diaspora communities strategise against it, in so doing, emboldening them to better advocate for their own health needs.

Works Cited

Aristotle. (1944). *Politics* (Vol. 1). (H. Rackham, Trans.). Harvard University Press. Retrieved June 2, 2022, from Perseus Catalogue: http://data.perseus.org/citations/urn:cts:greekLit:tlg0086.tlg035.perseus-eng1:1.1252b

Berwald, S., Roche, M., Adelman, N., & Livingstone, G. (2016). Black African and Caribbean British Communities' Perceptions of Memory Problems: "We Don't Do Dementia". *PLoS One, 11*(4). https://doi.org/10.1371/journal.pone.0151878

Braveman, P. A., Heck, K., Egerter, S., Marchi, K. S., Dominguez, T. P., Cubbin, C., et al. (2015). The Role of Socioeconomic Factors in Black-White Disparities in Preterm Birth. *American Journal of Public Health, 105*(4), 694–702.

BreastCancer.org. (2022, 7 25). https://www.breastcancer.org/risk/risk-factors/race-ethnicity. Retrieved from BreastCancer.org: https://www.breastcancer.org/risk/risk-factors/race-ethnicity

Clennon, O. D. (2019, February 22). *Research in Social Justice: Why "Whiteness" Matters in the Real World.* Retrieved June 1, 2022, from Palgrave Macmillan: https://www.palgrave.com/gp/campaigns/social-justice/ornette-clennon

Clennon, O. D. (2022, June 20). *Palgrave Studies in Decolonisation and Grassroots Black Organic Intellectualism (MaSPP).* Retrieved from MaCTRI (MEaP Academy Community Training and Research Institute): https://critracemmu.wordpress.com/decoloniality-in-the-grassroots-the-key-to-social-justice/

Demie, F. (2021). The Experience of Black Caribbean Pupils in School Exclusion in England. *Educational Review, 73*(1), 55–70.

Dzobo, N. K. (1992). African Symbols and Proverbs as Sources of Knowledge. In K. Wiredu & K. Gyekye (Eds.), *Person and Community: Ghanaian Philosophical Studies I (Vol. 1)* (pp. 85–98). Council for Research in Values and Philosophy.

Emeagwali, G. (2014). Intersections Between Africa's Indigenous Knowledge Systems and History. In G. Emeagwali & G. Sefa Dei (Eds.), *African Indigenous Knowledge and the Disciplines* (pp. 1–19). Sense Publishers.

Fenton, K., Pawson, E., & Souza-Thomas, L. (2020). *Beyond the Data: Understanding the Impact of COVID-19 on BAME Communities.* Public Health England. Available at https://assets.publishing.service.gov.uk/government/uploads/system/uploads/attachment_data/file/892376/COVID_stakeholder_engagement_synthesis_beyond_the_data.pdf.

GMCA. (2015, December 18). *Taking Charge of Our Health and Social Care in Greater Manchester.* Retrieved from GMCA: https://www.greatermanchester-ca.gov.uk/what-we-do/health/documents/

Gordon, L. (2009). *Black Intellectual Tradition.* Retrieved from Genius: https://genius.com/Lewis-gordon-black-intellectual-tradition-annotated

Gov.uk. (2019, July 25). *Permanent and Fixed Period Exclusions in England 2017 to 2018.* Retrieved from GOV.UK: https://www.gov.uk/government/statistics/permanent-and-fixed-period-exclusions-in-england-2017-to-2018

Gov.uk. (2021, January 1). *The NHS Constitution for England.* Retrieved from GOV.UK: https://www.gov.uk/government/publications/the-nhs-constitution-for-england/the-nhs-constitution-for-england#:~:text=constitution%2Dfor%2Dengland-,Introduction%20to%20the%20NHS%20Constitution,the%20end%20of%20our%20lives.

Gramsci, A. (1999). *Selections from the Prison Notebooks.* Electric Book Company.

Gyekye, K. (1995). *An Essay on African Philosophical Thought: The Akan Conceptual Scheme*. Temple University Press.

MacKinnon, D. (2015). Devolution, State Restructuring and Policy Divergence in the UK. *The Geographical Journal, 181*(1), 47–56.

Mantovani, N., Pizzolati, M., & Edge, D. (2017). Exploring the Relationship Between Stigma and Help-Seeking for Mental Illness in African-Descended Faith Communities in the UK. *Health Expectations, 20*(3), 373–384.

Marmot, M. (2010). *Strategic Review of Health Inequalities in England Post 2010: Marmot Review Final Report*. University College.

Marmot, M. (2020, February). *Health Equity in England: The Marmot Review 10 Years On*. Retrieved from The Health Foundation: https://www.health.org.uk/publications/reports/the-marmot-review-10-years-on

Mignolo, W. (2000). *Local Histories/Global Designs: Essays on the Coloniality of Power, Subaltern Knowledges and Border Thinking*. Princeton University Press.

Mignolo, W. (2002). The Geopolitics of Knowledge and the Colonial Difference. *South Atlantic Quarterly, 101*(1), 57–96.

Nazroo, J. Y., Falaschetti, E., Pierce, M., & Primatesta, P. (2009). Ethnic Inequalities in Access to and Outcomes of Healthcare: Analysis of the Health Survey for England. *Journal of Epidemiology and Community Health, 63*(12), 1022–1027.

NHS. (2022, 26 July). *NHS Long Term Plan*. Retrieved from NHS: https://www.longtermplan.nhs.uk/.

Pinder, R. J., Ferguson, J., & Møller, H. (2016). Minority Ethnicity Patient Satisfaction and Experience: Results of the National Cancer Patient Experience Survey in England. *BMJ Open, 6*(6) https://bmjopen.bmj.com/content/6/6/e011938

Pinto, R., Ashworth, M., & Jones, R. (2008). Schizophrenia in Black Caribbeans Living in the UK: An Exploration of Underlying Causes of the High Incidence Rate. *British Journal of General Practice, 58*(551), 429–434.

Rabiee, F., & Smith, P. (2014). Understanding Mental Health and Experience of Accessing Services Among African and African Caribbean Service Users and Carers in Birmingham, UK. *Diversity and Equality in Health and Care, 11*(2), 125–134.

Riches, N. (2016). *Black and Minority Ethnic Groups Health Needs Assessment*. Salford CVS. Available at https://www.salfordcvs.co.uk/sites/salfordcvs.co.uk/files/Salford%20BME%20Health%20Needs%20Assessment%202016.pdf. Retrieved from https://www.salfordcvs.co.uk/sites/salfordcvs.co.uk/files/Salford%20BME%20Health%20Needs%20Assessment%202016.pdf

Sefa Dei, G. (2014). Indigenizing the Curriculum: The Case of the African University. In G. Emeagwali & G. Sefa Dei (Eds.), *African Indigenous Knowledge and the Disciplines* (pp. 165–180). Sense Publishers.

Verhaeghe, P.-P., & Ghekiere, A. (2021). The Impact of the Covid-19 Pandemic on Ethnic Discrimination on the Housing Market. *European Societies, 23*(1), S384–S399.

Waghid, Y., & Smeyers, P. (2012). Reconsidering Ubuntu: On the Educational Potential of a Particular Ethic of Care. *Educational Philosophy and Theory, 44*(S2), 6–20.

Wallace, S., Nazroo, J., & Becares, L. (2016). Cumulative Effect of Racial Discrimination on the Mental Health of Ethnic Minorities in the United Kingdom. *American Journal of Public Health, 106*(7), 1294–1300.

Walshe, K., Coleman, A., McDonald, R., Lorne, C., & Munford, L. (2016). Health and Social Care Devolution: The Greater Manchester Experiment. *British Medical Journal (BMJ), 352.* https://doi.org/10.1136/bmj.i1495

Wellings, D. (2017, September 16). *What Does the Public Think About the NHS?* Retrieved from The King's Fund: www.kingsfund.org.uk/publications/what-does-publicthink-about-nhs

Wilson, C., Alam, R., Latif, S., Knighting, K., Williamson, S., & Beaver, K. (2012). Patient Access to Healthcare Services and Optimisation of Self-Management for Ethnic Minority Populations Living with Diabetes; A Systematic Review. *Health and Social Care in the Community, 20*(1), 1–19.

2

What Decoloniality Looks Like in the Health Market

Abstract In this chapter, using quality-adjusted life years (QALYs) as a case example, we will take a closer look at the disparities identified in Chap. 1 by examining the role of whiteness in Public Health and its impacts on African Diaspora health seekers. Using whiteness and its *historical patterns of behaviour* in forming "race", as an unethical framework and in essence decolonising whiteness, we will then examine the role and power of systems-gatekeepers in Public Health maintaining market failure for African Diaspora health seekers. In the final part of this chapter, we will also use the voices of community members to translate and ground the effect of systems-gatekeeping on their health and health-seeking behaviours.

Keywords Aristotelian human ethics • Gatekeepers in health • Coloniality of power • Whiteness

Introduction

Historical Formation of "Race"

We will take an ethical approach to examining the role of "race" in the formation of whiteness.

Firstly, we need to remember that today, whiteness is a societal ordering mechanism around power. Kamaljeet Gill, whilst exploring James Baldwin's film *I Am Not Your Negro* helpfully wrote that

> Whiteness is not a description of a race, it is rather a position in a power-relationship, which builds itself in opposition to all the people who are produced as not-white, and in particular those who are Black.

In *International Perspectives of Multiculturalism*, Clennon (2016) discusses how using a Fanonian lens (Fanon, 1963) to track how colonialism transformed into capitalism, we can see not-so-faint racial imprints ("coloniality of power" see Mignolo & Escobar, 2010; Mignolo, 2000) left behind by its colonial past. This means that although the current (cultural) market[1] is no longer necessarily defined by race, the positions of its market actors adopt template positions that used to be defined by racial loci. If we see whiteness as a *historical pattern of behaviour* (Clennon, 2019) that is primarily about defining a Western sense of identity through colonial expansion, we can see that this identity-forming process was first about religion and politics which very much became a proxy for proto-racialism via the process of Orientalism (see Said, 1978; Otele, 2020; Hall, 2009) of Dar al Islam (in opposition to Christendom). This early pattern of behaviour and superiority-complex led a fledgling Western identity to categorise people into human beings and non-human beings, firstly using religion (politics) as a measure of humanity (see

---

[1] See Clennon (2015) for a full discussion about how markets are formed and perform with Bourdesian and Foucauldian powers of institutions. Clennon also describes how culture, cultural memory and cultural narratives are commoditised and turned into Baudrillardian "sign values" for a consumer popular culture market, which finds material effect in the ethea of our governing institutions (Clennon, 2018).

Adib-Moghaddam, 2010; Santana, 2019; Hall, 2009). For us, it is important to locate colonialism and its ongoing coloniality within this historical framework of whiteness. So, we will examine whiteness in its three epochal stages; its conception, its gestation and its birth.

Let us first orientate whiteness within an ethical and moral framework as prescribed by Aristotle's "natural law" (Aristotle, 1944).

Aristotle and Non-human Slaves?

Decolonising Human Ethics

Santana (2019) gives a great break down of the Aristotelian concept of "natural slaves", where Aristotle thought that some people were naturally born to be slaves and others were born to be rulers. Aristotle outlined the hierarchical structures of his times by stating that Greeks were the apex of nobility (civility) and anyone outside that were barbarians. In Greek households, three partnerships (relationships) were deemed essential for a civil household: Mastery (over slaves), Marriage (with a woman) and Progeny (relationship with children).

However, in discussing Mastery, Aristotle believed that those who are naturally born with a nature to be enslaved are essentially property or animated tools of the Master (those born to "master") that enable him to carry out his daily tasks. However, it is important to note that for Aristotle slaves were still *human beings*, as they had the human traits of reason to recognise the will of their Master and to see that, as their own will. Aristotle believed that they understood reason but didn't possess it. We can interpret "reason" in this context to have a dual meaning in terms of using their own reason (will) to understand the reason (will) of their master but by being property they did not have the *agency* to assert their own reason (will). This is in distinct contrast to tamed animals who were deemed not to have any reason at all, just "feelings" ([1254b] [1] line 19). So, due to "reason", Aristotle believed that being a Master over a human slave (who also understands reason) was the highest calling ("function"

([1254a] [1] line 22)) in Greek society. However, Santana argues that Aristotle didn't see slaves as whole human beings because of their "lack" of reason but we would strongly disagree with this for the reasons just stated but also because Aristotle definitely believed in a human species with different types of natures within the species that prescribed different types of societal roles and different degrees of agency (such as master and slave):

> And the same must also necessarily apply in the case of mankind as a whole; therefore all men that differ as widely as the soul does from the body and the human being from the lower animal lines. [1254b] [1] lines 11–13

We would argue that even barbarians were thought of as human beings just a different type of human being in terms of their having "no class of natural rulers" (Aristotle, 1944, p. [1252b] [1] line 5), meaning supposedly having no agency of their own, bearing in mind that for Aristotle, only Greeks were naturally born rulers with agency. Concerning slaves, Aristotle says this himself:

> These considerations therefore make clear the nature of the slave and his essential quality: one who is a human being belonging by nature not to himself but to another is by nature a slave, and a person is a human being belonging to another if being a man he is an article of property, and an article of property is an instrument for action separable from its owner. [1254a] [1] lines 11–12

Aristotle also describes different classes of enslaved human beings when he writes about "slavery by law" ([1255a] [1] line 5) that produced captives from the vanquished who were then enslaved by the victors as being justifiable (by the law). Aristotle was more than aware of his detractors who argued against slavery during his time, even as he continued to propose that that class of slave was of a different sort to the "natural slaves". He explained that because "war-slaves" were made slaves by the law (agreement)[2] whereas "natural slaves" were made slaves by their nature, Greeks who became enslaved by war would still not be regarded as slaves as it wasn't in their nature!

Now, although the "natural slave" is the property of its owner, Aristotle shares an intriguing insight into the real status of the "natural slave":

and the slave is a part of the master—he is, as it were, a part of the body, alive but yet separated from it; hence there is a certain community of interest and friendship between slave and master in cases when they have been qualified by nature for those positions. [1255b] [1] lines 10–12

Aristotle is telling us that the "natural slave" is actually a part of the natural "master" without whom his household could not be run, whereas the "slave" might belong entirely to the "master", their worth exceeds their status of master's "slave". In a way, "this community of interest and friendship" implies a single unit of "reason" (for the household) comprising will (intention) and execution (turning intention into action). Within this unit of mastery, the master cannot master without execution, thus making the slave indispensable or the master at the slave's mercy! However,

---

[2] Very similar to some pre-colonial African attitudes towards slavery resulting from inter-ethnic rivalries. Diop (1987) gives a detailed account of the pre-colonial caste system in Senegal which he extrapolates as being typical across the Continent at that pre-colonial time. He describes how enslaved prisoners of war were supposed to be fully integrated into their new host communities. Diop describes how being assigned a slave to the Father's household or the Mother's household had significant implications for their societal trajectory. Interestingly, the lack of "community of interest" described by Aristotle between a slave by law and their master, in the Senegalese model, takes the form of the likelihood of the slave plotting and realising rebellion. This was less likely to happen if the slave was assigned to the Mother due to their child-rearing responsibilities and full integration into the domestic household. However, Diop explains that slaves assigned to the Father (who looked after administrative matters) were given special dispensation in terms of sharing the loot of raids and their proximity to power (patronage) via the King (Father), possibly to buy their loyalty as their positions were inherently precariously linked to the welfare of their Father, thus also making rebellion unlikely. Interestingly, Diop describes these slaves as slaves in name only, much like the Aristotelian slaves in law who did not consider themselves actual slaves (despite their positions). In Senegal, as a result of the status and designations, individuals of a higher rank (caste) were forbidden to mistreat slaves and were expected to assist them as much as they could, presumably to aid in community integration. What this brief Senegalese description shows is that slaves were not regarded as subhuman in the modern sense, with no human rights because pre-colonial slaves across the Ancient world were protected by intricate pre-colonial civil rights (or human ethics) granted to them by their communities/societies, as they were still considered human beings first and foremost.

Aristotle concedes that if the roles of master and slave are imposed by the law, such a harmonious relationship could not be guaranteed, as it would not be comprised of natural selves (especially in the case of a Greek slave under a barbarian master or even vice versa). So, for Aristotle, the *natural self* (which must mean the Ancient Grecian person)[3] was needed for both roles to operate symbiotically, causing the superficial facets of hierarchy to dissolve under this level of intense interdependence. Aristotle continues to describe this "somatic" relationship further:

> And the term 'article of property' is used in the same way as the term 'part': a thing that is a part is not only a part of another thing but absolutely belongs to another thing, and so also does an article of property. Hence whereas the master is merely the slave's master and does not belong to the slave, the slave is not merely the slave of the master but wholly belongs to the master.
> [1254a] [1] lines 7–10

This bears an uncanny resemblance to Hegel's (1977) *Phenomenology of the Spirit*, where he says that the Master gains his purpose from being a master of the slave, whereas the slave is not validated by the master but from his work, only. This will be explored later when discussing the relevance of this enquiry to a decolonial praxis.

So, Aristotle not only makes it clear that slaves are human beings albeit those with different "natures" (to rulers) they are indeed still human beings and if they are indeed part of the master and are indispensable to

---

[3] We can strongly infer this because Aristotle said "which implies that there are two kinds of nobility and of freedom, one absolute and the other relative" [1255a] [1] lines 29–30. For Aristotle, only Greeks had a universal (absolute) nobility that was "recognised" everywhere, whereas barbarian nobility could only be recognised locally (relative) in their region. Likewise, it was impossible for Greeks to be made slaves as captives via a "just war", but barbarians would always be slaves under these circumstances. In fact, Aristotle hints that if Greeks were to be taken captive and turned into slaves, they still could not be slaves because it could not have been a just war in the first place. So even though, undoubtedly, Aristotle believed in Grecian exceptionalism that placed Greeks by nature as the highest form of human being, even barbarians were considered human beings, albeit natural slaves. Reason being the quality attributed to human beings, whilst agency distinguishes the highest of human beings.

him with their *indispensable* value[4]—even to the extent of bestowing ultimate rank to their master and ruler:

for example to control a human being is a higher thing than to tame a wild beast. ([1254a] [1] line 21–22)

For us, to trace the "moral degeneracy" of dehumanising others to Aristotle is a little unfair, and yes this is a strong term because even for Aristotle, to first recognise the *humanity* of the "natural slave" was the highest accord of Greek civility where clearly, "taming a beast" (if ever slaves were thus considered) was not as highly esteemed.[5] Aristotle, as did many from the ancient, pre-colonial world, recognised ethnic differences and even formed complex social hierarchies based on these differences but with the distinct *ethical* position that recognised shared humanity, albeit from a Greco-centric perspective of top rank on the pyramid.[6]

---

[4] Aristotle (1944, pp. [1252a] [1] lines 21–28)

The first coupling together of persons then to which necessity gives rise is that between those who are unable to exist without one another… and the union of natural ruler and natural subject for the sake of security (for he that can foresee with his mind is naturally ruler and naturally master, and he that can do these things with his body is subject and naturally a slave; so that master and slave have the same interest).

[5] Robinson (1983) argues that Aristotle was not to be congratulated by this admission because he didn't go on to trace the exact qualities and value of slaves beyond their "nature". We agree with this but it still means that pre-modern ethics around slavery in Ancient Greece had an ethical sense of civil liberties within its own code of human ethics, in which different roles and their natures were considered. Also, for those who couldn't afford slaves, Aristotle says, "for the ox serves instead of a servant for the poor" (Aristotle, 1944, pp. [1252b] [1], line 11). They were obviously lower in societal status than those "controlling human beings".

[6] See Bernal (1987) and Diop (1974) for full discussions that locate African influences on ancient Greek culture and language. This is important because it underlines the fact that the Ancient pre-colonial world did not use ethnicity or race to dehumanise "others". "Others" were merely an "us and them" that was created by borders, conquests and alliances, language, and communication. Also see Diop (1987) in his *Comparative Study of the Political and Social Systems of Europe and Black Africa from Antiquity to the formation of Modern States* that also shows the pre-eminence of these pre-colonial human ethics that did not dehumanise.

The Myth of the Non-human

So why is this important?

Conception of Whiteness: Mapping the gradual loss of Human Ethics to Colonialism

To begin to witness the seeds of "dehumanisation", Heng (2018, p. 111) in reference to the Holy Crusades, writes that

> Though a number of names existed for the international enemy— Ishmaelites or Ismaelites, Agarenes or Hagarenes, Moors, Turks, Arabs, Persians, Ottomans, Mohammedans, and, in more general fashion, infidels, heathens, pagans, and even heretics—the preeminent name by which the enemy was known in Latin Europe for centuries was Saracens.

This is an important observation because of its contemporary echoes with the current homogeneity of "Blackness". Heng explains that Latin Europe (Latin referring to the then Catholic Church), categorised a diverse set of ethnic peoples who all practised Islam (which Latin Europe regarded as being based on a lie) into one homogenous block that was called the Saracens, which had an embedded meaning within it of "falseness" and "deviance". Once Latin Europe applied this intellectual sleight of hand, it became easier to attribute specific traits that demonised, if not dehumanised[7] them as an ethnic block. Heng (2018, p. 116) continues:

---

[7] In addressing this aspect of dehumanisation or loss of human ethics, Heng (2018, p. 118) writes about the multi-layered process of this loss that seems to have started during this period:

> Racialization of the Saracen is thus a multilayered phenomenon. At its most demonic—one might almost say ludic, or ludicrous—Saracens appear monstrous by being fused with animals, so that in the Chanson de Roland (Song of Roland) they have spiny bristles like a boar, or skin hard as iron, or they bark like dogs. No less damning, however, is to say that Muslims are monstrous in entirely human ways: that their "law" advocates unbridled, insensate lust and polymorphous perversity in this life and in the afterlife, monstrosifying human values.

To understand racial thinking, however, it is crucial to note that specific elements of the Prophet's imagined biography are imported into a general description of all Muslims, and thereafter assigned as the collective personality traits of those who share a common religion. Practices of generalization, through which the personality of a singular individual becomes transcoded into the character of a collective totality of peoples, exemplify processes of race thinking and racialization.

Heng regards this type of stereotyping (i.e. homogenisation and group labelling/essentialising) as a process of race thinking, even though built on religious bigotry at this point. It is also important to note that these ethnic groups did not return the favour of homogenisation or essentialising and still regarded their enemies in Christendom as fully fledged heterogenous ethnic human beings, "as "Romans, Greeks, Franks, Slavs," and so on" (Heng, 2018, p. 111).[8] However, from the "Saracens", we can see how the historical playbook of whiteness that homogenises and essentialises diverse ethnic peoples into a monolith can be applied to today's "Black" peoples (via the Negro). We can also definitely see how this is an important step towards dehumanisation, once cultural heritage and narrative are removed.[9] However, curiously Ibn Khaldûn, a fourteenth-century Arab scholar and sociologist (who would have been dubbed a Saracen), in his *The Muqaddimah* also noted the "invisibility" of this emerging whiteness in Mediaeval Europe, as he observed its tendency to categorise others:

> The inhabitants of the north are not called by their colour, because the people who established the conventional meanings of words were themselves white. Thus, whiteness was something usual and common to them, and they did not

---

[8] Implying that *their* pre-colonial human ethics were still intact.

[9] See Clennon (2018) for full discussion about how removing cultural and historical narratives about a diverse peoples in the name of political Blackness is unproductive and even plays into the hands of the racialising play book of whiteness.

see anything sufficiently remarkable in it to cause them to use it as a specific term. (Khaldûn, 2015, p. 86)[10]

---

[10] In his *The Muqaddimah*, Khaldûn made a distinct effort to understand the variations in the human species by discounting religious (Koranic) genealogies of race that hinted at the "natural slave": Genealogists who had no knowledge of the true nature of things imagined that Negroes were the children of Ham, the son of Noah, and that they were singled out to be black as the result of Noah's curse, which produced Ham's colour and the slavery God inflicted upon his descendants. (p. 85)

Instead Khaldûn sought more empirical explanations of differing skin colour and character, based on climate. Even when he observes:
We have seen that Negroes are in general characterized by levity, excitability, and great emotionalism. They are found eager to dance whenever they hear a melody. They are everywhere described as stupid. (p. 88)

Khaldûn himself is reluctant to denigrate the character of the Negro without proper empirical evidence:
Al-Mas'ûdî undertook to investigate the reason for the levity, excitability, and emotionalism in Negroes, and attempted to explain it. However, he did no better than to report, on the authority of Galen and Ya'qûb Ibn Isâq al Kindî, that the reason is a weakness of their brains which results in a weakness of their intellect. This is an inconclusive and unproven statement. (p. 89)

Khaldûn is reminding us that pre-colonial (i.e. non-Latin Europe) human ethics are still intact in the Mediaeval Arab world, although debated. In fact, more profoundly, Khaldûn is trying to use (climatic, ecological and habitat!) *empirism* to explain human differences rather than using religious or subjective processes more common to Mediaeval Europe at the time. It is also important to note that Khaldûn's use of "Negro" does not have the modern Robinsonian meaning of dehumanised African because his use describes specific peoples living in the distinct geographical areas according to his "scientific" (empirical) methods:
The inhabitants of the first and second zones in the south are called the Abyssinians, the Zanj, and the Sudanese. These are synonyms used to designate the particular nation that has turned black. The name 'Abyssinians', however, is restricted to those Negroes who live opposite Mecca and the Yemen, and the name 'Zanj' is restricted to those who live along the Indian Sea. These names are not given to them because of an alleged descent from a black human being, be it Ham or anyone else. Negroes from the south who settle in the temperate fourth zone or in the seventh zone that tends toward whiteness, are found to produce descendants whose colour gradually turns white in the course of time. Vice versa, inhabitants from the north or from the fourth zone who settle in the south produce descendants whose colour turns black. This shows that colour is conditioned by the composition of the air. (p. 86)

Even though according to Eze (1997) Immanuel Kant, as well as Linnaeus (1766) before him, also used the same (centuries old) environmental habitats-theory (or climatic determinism) to *determine* racial intellectual characteristics, we can safely say that neither Kant nor Linnaeus appeared to match the intellectual nuance of the mediaeval Arabic theorist Ibn Khaldûn, who himself, by using reason, resisted castigating the intellectual potential of Africans (because he wanted evidence) rather than succumbing to mere "feelings" (i.e. parroting "unproven statements" a.k.a. bigotries). And do remember that according to Aristotle, it was only wild beasts who were driven by their "feelings" as opposed to a "reason"-driven mankind as a whole!

Before briefly moving on to how the Valladolid debates used Aristotle's natural law to justify Spain's colonisation of the Americas, it is worth noting that Otele (2020) and Hall (2009) both copiously emphasise how an intact human ethic was applied to Africans in early Mediaeval Europe as trade delegations between the continents were lively and productive.[11]

Gestation of Whiteness: Valladolid and Natural Law: Loss of Human Ethics?

In the 1550 Valladolid debates, between Las Casas and Sepúlveda about whether to enslave the native Amerindians they had encountered, we can see how the Aristotelian concept of the "natural slave" was applied. Brunstetter & Zartner (2011) give a good account of the opposing positions of these arguments. Sepúlveda (2021) deliberately chose to discount the hallmarks of civilisation that the Spanish had encountered and

---

[11] Hall (2009, p. 1) reminds us that:

Before the Atlantic slave trade began, racism justifying slavery in medieval Spain and Portugal was aimed at people with light skin. Although there were some enslaved blacks there, slave status was identified with whites. The very word "slave" is derived from "Slav": whites who were captured in Eastern Europe and shipped into medieval Spain in large numbers. Racist ideology was based on climatic determinism, but it was the Slavs who were considered natural slaves.

labelled them savage because of their religious customs.[12] There is a sense of "moral degeneracy" manifesting in the form of hypocrisy that we describe creeping in here because although Sepúlveda acknowledges their civilisational achievements (some of which even seem to echo democracy—understood only from our present-day vantage point—i.e. "non-hereditary kings who are elected by popular suffrage" [para. 3]) and that they are "neither bears nor monkeys and that they are not totally irrational" (Sepúlveda, 2021, para. 3). So, Sepúlveda is definitely *implying* and acknowledging their inherent humanity), he still manages to dismiss them, as savages (natural slaves) in order to undergird his thesis of an Aristotelian "just war" of conquest.

On the other hand, Las Casas specifically and directly appealed to their *inherent* humanity (meaning an Aristotelian "mankind as a whole") via his Catholic beliefs of their not being created as beasts. And with their innate humanity they were capable of being converted to Catholicism, in the process of being spared slavery (encomienda) (Pharo, 2014). The

---

[12] In summary, Sepúlveda (2021) argued from his 1571 treatise, *The Second Democrates* that the indigenous Amerindians although not devoid of reason were still savages due to their "barbarous institutions and customs" even though:

> They boast of their political and social institutions, because they have rationally planned cities and nonhereditary kings who are elected by popular suffrage, and they carry on commerce among themselves in the manner of civilized people. (para. 3)

In this instance, he follows Aristotle clearly by recognising their nobility (and "reason") but that it is local rather than universal (absolute), meaning for Sepúlveda that their inherent slave natures (as illustrated by their violent pagan customs) made them ripe for conquering. Even their feudal system had them tarnished as natural slaves in Sepúlveda's eyes, despite the Spanish feudal system itself only fully ending in 1820! (Delmar, 1875). However, see Kosto (2011) for a full discussion about historians' uncertainty about which regions of Spain were under feudal control and for how long and whether the terms of reference for feudalism had changed over time. The irony of Sepúlveda's hypocrisy is magnified even further in the context of Spain's own brutal religious persecutions and murders under the Spanish Inquisition (1478–1834) where the ecclesiastical class as led by the Grand Inquisitors (e.g. Tomás de Torquemada who was the first Grand Master and who was famous for his extreme brutality) protected the religious purity of the Spanish Crown by converting or ethnically cleansing Muslims and Jews from their regions. It is interesting but not surprising that he failed to see the parallels between his own country and that of the indigenous people who also lived under symbiotically entwined religious and ruling classes. Spanish murderous brutality for their God was "civilised" but of course, indigenous sacrificing for theirs, was not! We call this moral blindness, the *Sepúlveda complex*, which will be pointed out throughout the volume, as it re-appears in different guises.

Spanish Courts seemed to side with Las Casas in the end.[13] However, for us, what is interesting was Sepúlveda's inherent understanding of their humanity (even listing their civilisational achievements) despite his stringent desire to make them "slaves by law", as Aristotle had described. So even though Sepúlveda saw the indigenous people as "slaves by nature" (primarily because of their religious practices and their serfdom) and inherent human beings, he still felt that they needed to be subdued by force in order to attain Spanish civility.[14] To add more ambiguity to their supposed barbarian status and land ownership (that Sepúlveda sneered at because of their communitarian landownership practice), the Spanish government still had to account in law for the conflict between prior indigenous ownership of the land and the Spanish Crown's rights of ownership. Saavedra (2020, p. 226) explains how the Spanish managed to reconcile these opposing types of land ownership by making a distinction between private and public law (in Roman law), where private law acknowledges indigenous pre-existing ownership of the land:

> The state, he [José María Mariluz Urquijo] argued, was the only owner of lands in America, but this ownership was only considered eminent domain or sovereignty and not property in terms of private law .... This sleight of hand not only neatly reconciled both arguments discussed above, but it also went further by recognizing private property as the only manner of land tenure in Spanish America—irrespective of if it meant indigenous or Spanish property.

So, although at this very time in Spain, the concept of "race" as a dehumanising tool was not (quite) aimed at the indigenous of the Americas, we can definitely see that it was explicitly aimed at ethnically cleansing Jewish communities living in Spain. Nirenberg (2014, p. 248) tells us that:

---

[13] See Alva (1991) in his *Colonizing Souls* who provides an excellent description of how the Spanish Inquisition when transported to the Americas had to transform its methods of physical brutality (thanks to Las Casas' recommendations) into a more psychological and ethnographical form of conversion.

[14] Remember that Aristotle thought that making slaves by the law was an unharmonious option for the slave/master model as there would not be a "community of interest" between the roles.

Already in the early fifteenth century "raza," "casta" and "linaje" (race, caste, lineage) were part of a complex of closely associated terms that linked both behavior and appearance to nature and reproduction. Some of these words, like the word "lineage" itself, had long been used to tie character to genealogy, and the history of that usage was largely independent of "Jewish" questions.

However, we can more clearly see the first signs of "raza" (race) as a specific tool of dehumanisation, here and we must remember that it was first reserved for Jewish communities:

The Castilian word "raza," however, was much newer, and it seems to have come into broad usage as a term in the animal and the human sciences more or less simultaneously. Although the earliest use I know of in Castilian deploys the term to refer to a hoof disease in horses, among breeders the word "raza" quickly came to mean, in the first quarter of the fifteenth century, something like "pedigree." (Nirenberg, 2014, p. 248)

So, now we can see a progression towards an unethical dehumanising of fellow human beings as epitomised by the words Saracen (Islamophobia), savage (Indigenous Indians) and "raza" (Anti-Semitism) that through the religious bigotries of Christendom (proto-whiteness as observed by Ibn Khaldûn) all laid the foundations for a fully blown concept of race that later became exclusively associated with African-ness and non-human-ness. But we can definitely see from the perspective of Aristotle and the wider Ancient world that this is a perversion of the "natural law" that helped to defined human ethics at *and* of the time.

The Birth of Whiteness: What's the non-human African got to do with it?

So far, we have taken the time to reflect on the historical hallmarks of whiteness from its conception to gestation. We have also identified how early forms of whiteness used tools of mastery to denigrate others (particularly Muslims, Jews and Indigenous Americans) as they gradually departed from the Aristotelian and wider Ancient world (including

Mediaeval Arab) human ethics[15] based on human "reason" and coopera-tion[16] under "natural law". We did this to provide a pre-colonial context for human ethics with its discussions, debates and transformations over time.

Whiteness and Capitalism

In his *Black Marxism*, Robinson (1983) writes about how Europe devel-oped "race" as an instrument of subjection that initially was turned inwards upon itself before being applied to Africans. In *Black Scholarly Activism*, Clennon (2018) argued that it was "ethnicity" rather than "race" that was being used in this way and that it only turned into race with the advent of a capitalism that was built on and by slavery. We would, however, like to correct that view having traced the seeds of the concept of "race" and its unethical applications over the centuries. So, what the Transatlantic Slave trade brought wasn't a particularly new idea of race, per se or a system of racism (racial law, racial contract, see Mills, 1997 and scientific racism, see Linnaeus, 1766), but a fully fledged white-ness that had already developed those tools of subjugation from its con-ception to gestation, as we have outlined.

This means that Robinson's description of how the enslaved African was stripped of all historicity and homogenised[17] into a Negro without history or provenance but with definite negative traits[18] that now are

---

[15] It is important that throughout our discussions about the emergence of whiteness that we have been using a connected histories framework of critical enquiry. See Bhambra (2010) and Bhambra (2007).

[16] Remembering that slaves under Aristotelian "natural law" worked harmoniously as "a part of the body" of their Master for the running of his household. Also remembering the Senegalese analogue of this, as described by Diop that prescribed "slavery" as an integrative and legal process of assimi-lating foreigners into existing kinship networks (with the political implications that process brought with it, depending on their patron).

[17] Remember the creation of the "Saracens"; essentialising a diverse set of people within their homogenisation.

[18] Remember Sepúlveda's attempts to do this to the indigenous peoples he encountered in the Americas.

explicitly racialised[19] as non-human, is really a description about the *birth* of whiteness, its modus operandi and the extent of its "moral degeneracy". Many scholars (e.g. Andrews, 2021; Hall, 2009; Williams, 1994; Otele, 2020; Gilroy, 1993; Gopal, 2019, etc.) have written at great length about how the industrial need for slave labour for the cotton and sugar plantations across imperial domains created the need for a dehumanised African unit of labour. So, we don't need to rehearse well-known arguments and analyses, here. But we think it is important to state that aside from the brutal treatment of slaves[20] and their numerous rebellions for freedom,[21] the specific "moral degeneracy" of whiteness and its *birth* at this time, was that it completely broke away from any form of pre-colonial human ethics (i.e. the valuing of "mankind as whole" as human) in order to create an unfettered path to pursue profit (from Black bodies). In other words, its "moral degeneracy" is directly linked to and even embedded in this modern world system we call capitalism that was built by global imperialism (Fanon, 1963).[22] In the next section we will track how the historical hallmarks of whiteness that we have just identified underpin and shape access to the health market for Black health seekers.

The Role of Whiteness in the Health Market

The ethical and moral aspect of whiteness is particularly relevant to the health market because there are only finite and limited resources. Also, where questions about who is prioritised (or neglected) emerge, especially from an ethical viewpoint, tracing the conception and development of whiteness into colonialism (see Chap. 3), and then capitalism becomes an urgent priority.

---

[19] Remember "raza" as a measure of pedigree of animals, specifically applied to Jews.

[20] Remember brutal violence is what demoted the indigenous peoples in the Americas to the status of savage.

[21] These are the extreme consequences of making people "slaves by law", although in this instance they weren't seen as people.

[22] See Clennon (2016) for a psychoanalytical reading of how the pathology of male-gendered whiteness acts as a derivative for markets in a neoliberal paradigm. This chapter's outlining of the origins of whiteness acting very much as a companion piece for whiteness' fundamental role in shaping neoliberal markets.

One overlooked aspect of whiteness in healthcare lies within health economics. The notion of whiteness in this context only has meaning through the construction of Blackness, or as Robinson would call it, The Negro. And for us, this is what lies as the basis for whiteness in the health market, where whiteness is construed as being treated as a human being.

The Invisibility of Whiteness

The inhabitants of the north are not called by their colour, because the people who established the conventional meanings of words were themselves white. Thus, whiteness was something usual and common to them, and they did not see anything sufficiently remarkable in it to cause them to use it as a specific term. (Khaldûn, 2015, p. 86)

The white body continues to be seen as the standard template for assessing health needs, which lies with the National Institute of Care Excellence (NICE) and the quality-adjusted life years (QALYs), about both of which we will speak later. Here, it is whiteness that is the biological template in the medical model upon which many priority treatments and interventions are based. We refer to this practice as "benchmarking" because this is the standard measure (where the common denominator is white) that is used to determine practices and to where resources are directed. For example, the widely used pulse oximeter used to assess and detect blood oxygen levels does not take into account the pigment in dark skin. Although this tool was highlighted as unreliable in 2020, we already knew about the biased results from pulse oximeters because they were identified in a research paper over 30 years ago by Jubran and Tobin (1990). However, this measure continues to be deemed an efficient way for spotting signs in deteriorating individuals in clinical incidences such as those with COVID-19, even though we know it gives biased and unreliable results for people with darker skin! So, we can see that the continued use of the pulse oximeter effectively deprioritises the Black body because despite knowledge of its bias, it continues to be used with the consequence of potentially delaying Black individuals being referred for the care needed to prevent further health deterioration.

Here is another example of benchmarking the white body (in this case, the white male body) that one of our community partners has experienced:

> It is ridiculous that Black people are still not being offered screening for prostate cancer until they are 50 years old. My brother who is in his mid-40's visited the GP with problems passing urine. He had been a couple of times over the last few months with the same complaint and it was only on the 3rd visit that the GP decided to offer him an examination for prostate cancer despite my brother telling the GP that my dad died early from prostate cancer.

Gatekeeping and Whiteness

In the UK, the use of drugs and of resources is based upon decisions that assess the "cost-effectiveness" (i.e. cost vs. benefits) of an intervention. The "effectiveness" of a treatment is often determined by a metric known as the quality-adjusted life year (QALY), which assigns a financial value to patients in relation to an intended treatment. However, we believe that the QALY is not the best tool for decision making because it does not address equity concerns for the Black health seeker. We can see this particularly when we think about the link between racism and rare diseases. For example, our community partners (from both African and Caribbean backgrounds) often talk about Sickle Cell disease[23] as a debilitating condition. They cannot understand the ignorance displayed around this condition in healthcare. Knowledge of Sickle Cell (remember, the most commonly inherited blood disorder in Black communities [populations]) continues to be deprioritised in terms of treatment, education and work when compared to cystic fibrosis which is commonly recognised as an illness that predominantly affects white communities (populations).

---

[23] NHS (2022, paras 3, 4)

> People with sickle cell disease produce unusually shaped red blood cells that can cause problems because they do not live as long as healthy blood cells and can block blood vessels.

> Sickle cell disease is a serious and lifelong health condition, although treatment can help manage many of the symptoms.

Decision makers, who are often white do not have a lived experience of some of the rare conditions such as Sickle Cell, so attach fewer resources for treatment or even human resources (including education of nurses and medics) despite the significant costs to the Black individual in terms of quality of life.

A community partner put this into tragic context for us:

> Ten days later mum started having pains rang the hospital several times only to find out she was haemorrhaging and needed a blood transfusion. The sad thing here is that even though they knew she had sickle before arrival, they could not get the blood match, we then lost a mother.

Overall, the life expectancy of Black people, due to racism and discrimination is lower than that of their white counterparts and what is referred to as weathering,[24] forces Black people to have more ill health. So, the QALY is used as a generalised cost-effective measure without taking into account Black people who experience more disadvantage. It does not take into account the psychosocial impact of those weathering factors that create barriers and stop Black people from fulfilling their full potential. In QALY terms, this translates to Black people being deemed more difficult to treat.

Another example, we cite, is that during the height of the pandemic Black people shared fears about being victims of COVID-19 and ending up in hospital. They were concerned about the de-prioritisation of Black people for ventilation or intensive care due to the underlying health issues that Black people often have (due to weathering), where this would deny them access to priority treatments, as based on quality measures made by mainly white decision makers. Tracking the hallmarks of whiteness, in this way can help us to understand how the market is set up for health and how important control is for operations at leadership levels.

---

[24] Forrester et al. (2019) describe weathering as accelerated biological ageing (e.g. internal "wear and tear" leading to higher prevalence of cardiovascular disease) in Black populations, due to exposure to racism and its psychosocial effects. Coogan et al. (2020) also link "wear and tear" to dementia and report how experiences of racism can increase the probability of developing it in later years.

Saracenisation: Homogenising and Essentialising

Black women in our communities speak about how they have been subject to dehumanisation in maternity care where they have been treated as second-class citizens, being ignored, disrespected and essentialised as "angry Black women" when in pain and in need of care and compassion. In our community conversations, Black women often speak about the unwillingness of some midwives to even touch them, which at the time, obviously denied them the humanity and dignity they deserved as human beings.

One of our community partners told us:

> I could not get over the way the midwife ignored me when I rung the buzzer for help after my caesarean section … it was like … I couldn't believe it, the buzzer was going and I thought she came to help me but walked straight past me and went to help the White lady who wasn't even ringing for assistance … I felt so undervalued, I felt like nothing … ahh.

In our conversations, the women often describe the feeling of the hurt of exclusion, especially when their new-born babies are already subjected to racism by also not receiving the care that they need. This process of dehumanisation produces a double disadvantage and devaluation of Black women based on their race and gender because there is a perception of Black women that deems them to be strong, sexualised and/or aggressive. See Chap. 3 for more about how race and gender for both Black women and Black men have been shaped by imperial whiteness, its relationship to intersectionality and its modern-day consequences for health.

So overall, we can see how the QALY acts as an instrument of whiteness, as it distorts human ethics (as implied by Aristotle) by placing a lower value on people's lives due to having less "life years" or "perfect health" ahead of them. As we can also see, this is a particular issue for Black people, since QALYs dictate that worth is *proportionate* to life expectancy.

> Homogenising us and treating us like animals. ("raza")

Here our community partners talk about being "Saracenised" and how they feel they have been treated like animals according to echoes of the "raza" and its (original) determination of animal pedigree:

> It is so upsetting and devaluing, I have been so unhappy at times with how I have been treated as a second-class citizen when I ask for information. I am often ignored, I mean, I am there physically but you can just tell by their body language and facial expressions that they have no interest in what you are asking which I guess wouldn't happen if I was White. It is like they see you as underserving.

One of the women that had had a hysterectomy said:

> I can honestly say that I did not get half the time that I see others getting with the nurses. When I was being discharged, I could hear all of the explanations being given to the woman behind the next curtain to me but when it came to me being discharged by the same nurse it was so quick and I was given so much less information about what to do if … I was treated as lesser than the other White woman.

The issue of care and how Black people are treated come up in many of our community conversations and we often take the opportunity to introduce them to the book *The Immortal Life of Henrietta Lacks* by Rebecca Skloot (Skloot, 2011). The book charts the true story of a poor Black woman Henrietta Lacks and highlights her mistreatment and betrayal by the medical profession, as she attended a poor charity-hospital in America. The medical profession stole and sold her cancerous cervical cells to research without her consent when she was diagnosed with cervical cancer.[25]

One of our community partners wanted to express how the book made her feel about the persistent mistreatment and devaluation of Black people, especially Black women.

> I was handed this book some-time ago and read it and was so angry in how they portrayed Henrietta in their usual racist ways as this Black strong loose woman and mother of five who had no idea of how to look after and

---

[25] See Chap. 3 for similar unethical behaviour towards Black men in the Tuskegee experiments.

respect her own body. This is similar to all those other experiments when they test on us Black people like animals.

This feeling of being treated like animals persists in our communities, as our partners often describe real-life scenarios such as when their blood cannot be matched. Our partners tell us that they innately or even subliminally do not necessarily trust the system in the sense of are people from their communities going to directly benefit from it, for instance, are they actually giving blood, and is it actually going to be used? Compounding their fears, they also cite health scares in the past where haemophiliacs had contracted the AIDS virus and Hepatitis C via blood transfusions.[26] So, our communities remain very protective and very self-preserving. See Chap. 3 for more details about the impact imperial whiteness and its Sepúlveda complex has had on historically shaping this mistrust.

Conclusion

In this chapter, we have traced the unethical emergence of whiteness over the longue durée, and we have briefly described how its historical patterns of behaviour underpin the actions of today's health market and its gatekeepers. In the next chapter, we will drill down into more detail about how whiteness and its imperial stages of development continue to affect the life opportunities of Black women and Black men in the UK and how it shapes their inequitable access to the health market.

Works Cited

Adib-Moghaddam, A. (2010). *A Metahistory of the Clash of Civilisations: Us and THEM BEYOND ORIENTALISm*. Hurst; Columbia University Press.
Alva, J. K. (1991). One – Colonizing Souls: The Failure of the Indian Inquisition and the Rise of Penitential Discipline. In M. E. Perry, & A. J. Cruz (Eds.),

---

[26] See BBC News (2022) for more details.

Cultural Encounters: The Impact of the Inquisition in Spain and the New World. https://publishing.cdlib.org/ucpressebooks/view?docId=ft396nb1 w0&chunk.id=d0e170&toc.depth=1&toc.id=d0e170&brand=ucpress. University of California Press. Retrieved from UC Press E-Books Collection, 1982–2004: https://publishing.cdlib.org/ucpressebooks/view?docId=ft396 nb1w0;brand=ucpress

Andrews, K. (2021). *The New Age of Empire: How Racism and Colonialism Still Rule the World.* Bold Type Books.

Aristotle. (1944). *Politics* (Vol. 1). (H. Rackham, Trans.). Harvard University Press. Retrieved June 2, 2022, from Perseus Catalogue: http://data.perseus. org/citations/urn:cts:greekLit:tlg0086.tlg035.perseus-eng1:1.1252b

BBC News. (2022, June 27). *Sir John Major Calls Contaminated Blood Scandal 'Incredibly Bad Luck'.* Retrieved from BBC News: https://www.bbc.co.uk/news/health-61929986

Bernal, M. (1987). *Black Athena The Afroasiatic Roots of Classical Civilization.* Rutgers University Press.

Bhambra, G. K. (2007). *Rethinking Modernity: Postcolonialism and the Sociological Imagination.* Palgrave Macmillan.

Bhambra, G. K. (2010). Historical Sociology, International Relations and Connected Histories. *Cambridge Review of International Affairs, 23*(1), 127–143.

Brunstetter, D. R., & Zartner, D. (2011). Just War Against Barbarians: Revisiting the Valladolid Debates Between Sepúlveda and Las Casas. *Political Studies, 59*(3), 733–752.

Clennon, O. (2015). *Urban Dialectics, The Market and Youth Engagement.* Nova Science Publishers. Available at https://www.academia.edu/15757142/Urban_Dialectics_The_Market_and_Youth_Engagement_The_Black_Face_of_Eurocentrism

Clennon, O. D. (2016). The Black Face of Eurocentrism: Uncovering Globalisation. In O. D. Clennon (Ed.), *International Perspectives of Multiculturalism: The Ethical Challenges* (pp. 91–128). Nova Science Publishers.

Clennon, O. D. (2018). *Black Scholarly Activism Between the Academy and Grassroots: A Bridge for Identities and Social Justice.* Palgrave Macmillan.

Clennon, O. D. (2019, February 22). *Research in Social Justice: Why "Whiteness" Matters in the Real World.* Retrieved June 1, 2022, from Palgrave Macmillan: https://www.palgrave.com/gp/campaigns/social-justice/ornette-clennon

Coogan, P., Schon, K., Li, S., Cozier, Y., Bethea, T., & Rosenberg, L. (2020). Experiences of racism and subjective cognitive function in African American women. *Alzheimer's & Dementia: Diagnosis, Asessment & Disease, 12*(1), e12067 https://doi.org/10.1002/dad2.12067. Retrieved from Alzheimer's Association.

Delmar, A. (1875). The Resources, Productions and Social Condition of Spain. *Proceedings of the American Philosophical Society, 14*(94), 301–343.

Diop, C. A. (1974). *The African Origin of Civilization: Myth or Reality.* (M. Cook, Ed., & M. Cook, Trans.). Lawrence Hill Books/Chicago Review Press.

Diop, C. A. (1987). *Pre-colonial Black Africa: Comparative Study of the Political and Social Systems of Europe and Black Africa from Antiquity to the Formation of Modern States.* (H. J. Salemson, Trans.). Lawrence Hill and Company.

Eze, E. C. (Ed.). (1997). *Post Colonial African Philosophy: A Reader.* Blackwell Publishers.

Fanon, F. (1963). The Wretched of the Earth. (C. Farrington, Trans.). Grove Press.

Forrester, S., Jacobs, D., Zmora, R., Schreiner, P., Roger, V., & Kiefe, C. I. (2019). Racial Differences in Weathering and Its Associations with Psychosocial Stress: The CARDIA Study. *SSM - Population Health, 7.* Available at https://www.sciencedirect.com/science/article/pii/S2352827318302246#:~:text=W eathering%20(W)%20was%20defined%20as,biologically%20younger%20 than%20their%20CA

Gilroy, P. (1993). *The Black Atlantic: Modernity and Double-Consciousness.* Verso.

Gopal, P. (2019). *Insurgent Empire: Anticolonial Resistance and British Dissent.* Verso.

Hall, G. M. (2009). *Slavery and African Ethnicities in the Americas: Restoring the Links.* The University of North Carolina Press.

Hegel, G. (1977). *The Phenomenology of Spirit.* (A. V. Miller, Trans.). Clarendon Press.

Heng, G. (2018). *The Invention of Race in the Middle Ages.* Cambridge University Press.

Jubran, A., & Tobin, M. J. (1990). Reliability of Pulse Oximetry in Titrating Supplemental Oxygen Therapy in Ventilator-Dependent Patients. *Chest Journal, 97*(6), 1420–1425.

Khaldûn, I. (2015). *The Muqaddimah: An Introduction to History.* (N. J. Dawood, Ed., & F. Rosenthal, Trans.). Princeton University Press.

Kosto, A. J. (2011). What About Spain? Iberia in the Historiography of Medieval European Feudalism. In S. Bagge, M. H. Gelting, & T. Lindkvist (Eds.), *FEUDALISM: New Landscapes of Debate* (pp. 135–159). Brepols Publishers.

Linnaeus, C. (1766). *Systema Naturae Ed. 12, Vol. 1.* Retrieved June 8, 2022, from The Linnean Collections: https://linnean-online.org/119981/#?s=0&cv=4

Mignolo, W. (2000). *Local Histories/Global Designs: Essays on the Coloniality of Power, Subaltern Knowledges and Border Thinking*. Princeton University Press.

Mignolo, W. D., & Escobar, A. (Eds.). (2010). *Globalization and the Decolonial Option*. Routledge.

Mills, C. W. (1997). *The Racial Contract*. Cornell University Press.

NHS. (2022, April 16). *Overview: Sickle Cell Disease*. Retrieved from NHS: https://www.nhs.uk/conditions/sickle-cell-disease/#:~:text=People%20 with%20sickle%20cell%20disease,manage%20many%20of%20the%20 symptoms

Nirenberg, D. (2014). *Neigboring Faiths: Christianity, Islam and Judaism in the Middle Ages and Today*. University of Chicago Press.

Otele, O. (2020). *African Europeans: An Untold History*. Hurst & Company.

Pharo, L. K. (2014). The Council of Valladolid (1550–1551): A European Disputation About the Human Dignity of Indigenous Peoples of the Americas. In M. Düwell, J. Braarvig, R. Brownsword, & D. Mieth (Eds.), *The Cambridge Handbook of Human Dignity Interdisciplinary Perspectives* (pp. 95–100). Cambridge University Press.

Robinson, C. (1983). *Black Marxism: The Making of the Black Radical Tradition*. Zed Press.

Saavedra, M. B. (2020). The Normativity of Possession. Rethinking Land Relations in Early-Modern Spanish America, ca. 1500–1800. *Colonial Latin American Review, 29*(2), 223–238.

Said, E. (1978). *Orientalism*. Vintage Books.

Santana, A. (2019). "The Indian Problem" Conquest and the Valladolid Debate. In R. E. Sanchez (Ed.), *Latin American and Latinx Philosophy: A Collaborative Introduction* (p. 290). Routledge.

Sepúlveda, J. G. (2021). *Democrates Alter Sive de Justis Belli Causis Apud Indos 1547*. Retrieved June 6, 2022, from Digital Histories: https://www.digital-history.uh.edu/active_learning/explorations/spain/spain_sepulveda.cfm

Skloot, R. (2011). *The Immortal Life of Henrietta Lacks*. Broadway Books.

Williams, E. (1994). *Capitalism and Slavery*. University of North Carolina Press.

3

The Racial and Gendered Determinants of Health

Abstract In this chapter, we will track the early development of whiteness to its imperial stages. Using a conversation between the authors and commentaries with contributions from community partners, we will uncover the impact that whiteness' *historical patterns of behaviour* has had on their lives. We believe that this needs to be fully acknowledged in order to really understand the daily experiences of African Diaspora health seekers and the (whiteness-induced) social stressors that ultimately lead to lower health outcomes. We will then briefly historically locate Bourdieu's, (1977) social and cultural capitals in whiteness and its imperial patriarchal structures, with their effect on the ability of the African Diaspora health seeker to benefit equitably from the health market.

Finally, we will examine Crenshaw's (1991) intersectionality within the framework of imperial whiteness and explore its suitability as a sufficiently inclusive framework that can help us to understand the relationships between Black Masculinities and Black male health-seeking behaviours, alongside its use to examine the inequalities of health outcomes for Black women.

Keywords Whiteness • Empire • Gender • Intersectionality • Coloniality of power • Gender

© The Author(s), under exclusive license to Springer Nature Switzerland AG 2022   **39**
F. Bruce, O. D. Clennon, *Decolonising Public Health through Praxis*,
https://doi.org/10.1007/978-3-031-18405-5_3

Introduction

Inspired by bell hook's and Cornel West's, *Breaking Bread: Insurgent Black Intellectual Life*, [1] we thought that the best way to break down these ideas about whiteness and intersectionality would be to explore them through a conversation about our backgrounds growing up as a Black British woman and a Black British man in the UK, as they relate to our experiences of health seeking.

Coloniality of Power: Resisting Whiteness

Ornette: Faye, in our numerous conversations about this, I remember you saying "something just didn't seem right from my childhood through to adulthood—neglect". What did you mean by this?

Faye: Well, I was born to Jamaican parents who migrated to England in 1961, they left Jamaica in search of a time limited opportunity that would make them enough money to send back to Jamaica and to return there with better prospects. My mum and dad came together as a couple, ended up getting married and still together 61 years later.

O: My grandparents were the same and were followed over by my mother and father. Wow, congrats to them on their 61 years together. My grandparents are also still together but my parents divorced when I was very young.

F: Throughout my adulthood I have reflected a lot about my life as a child growing up to Jamaican parents living in a predominantly white area of the city. Unconsciously there was always the feeling of difference and lack of acceptance, which started early in my childhood and made me unhappy for many reasons. I spent many mornings crying at the infant school gates as my mum or godmother left me there for the school day. I was reminded in many ways (by my all-white teachers) how useless they really thought I was. How humiliating as I think back to how teachers picked on me to answer questions and when I did not know the answer one teacher looked at me and asked "what is the matter with you people?"

---

[1] See hooks and West (1999).

O: At my school, I knocked around with a group of boys who were sick of being docked marks from their work for no reason. So, we were dubbed the one-percent boys because we would challenge the teachers asking them why they had marked our work incorrectly in terms of saying that our answers were wrong when the same answers from other white children were marked as correct! I think this also came about because our teachers had already consigned us to the rubbish heap of academic achievement.

F: Even though I mixed with those from different racial backgrounds I stood out I knew I was different, especially when it came to activities outside of school. For years, I blamed it on my parents and said it was unfair that I was never allowed to go to children's parties and other children's houses but, it was not about my parents excluding me from socialising and building social networks, it was the white parents that prevented this from happening.

O: Wow! That is crazy that you were actually experiencing what in effect was bullying (via exclusion) from the white parents of your friends! My bullying remained at school with the teachers, predominantly as my one-percent clique was a multicultural bunch (Afro Caribbean, Pakistani, White working class and Jewish)

Working twice as hard ....

O: Can you remember what your parents would say to you during these awful times?

F: Yes, I am reminded of some of my mother's strongest and most compelling stories whilst growing up. I always remember mum using her own experiences and that of her friends since arriving in the UK to tell me that as a Black woman I had to work twice as hard as White people throughout my education to achieve success. I always remember mum saying, "if they get a 'B', then you need to get an 'A' plus".

O: Yup. I remember my mum saying something similar, "you very well know that you have to be ten times better than your white friends ... So, why aren't you doing your homework?"

F: The magnitude of what this meant and how widespread this saying was within my communities made me believe that there was some truth in this and therefore eventually when I had finished, school conditioned me to adapt my own beliefs to try and succeed. However, working twice as hard to get just as far did not mean that Black people reached the goal that they aspired to achieve ... in fact many people did not. Whilst researching this, I came to realise that although this saying is predominantly widespread within American literature, this aphorism was also a commonly held principle that identified education as the key to equality and respectability, hence the 'work harder' ethic and the "Politics of Respectability".[2]

O: Yes, this old chestnut, 'if only we work hard enough, we will be accepted'. The Politics of Respectability is a busted flush, in my opinion because it responsibilises us for the systemic oppression we face, where in reality our efforts are certainly not effective in convincing the system to stop oppressing us. I guess at that time, though this was the only way that our folks could imagine a way out of this hell.

F: Yes, indeed there was an expectation from my parents that I remained strong, persevered and set my aspirations high so that I did not endure the hardship that they and their friends had encountered when they came to live in the UK in the 1960s.

O: Same. My mum always expected me to go to university even when I had other ideas of wanting to go to music college (due to aspirations of wanting to become a professional classical musician). She said gaining a university degree would open more doors for me. Looking back on it, she wasn't wrong!!

Commentary

The remnants of colonialism are everywhere as it is embedded in our institutions and in their patterns of behaviour. But if we remember Chap. 2, these patterns of behaviour are older than colonialism but still nevertheless, contribute to the wider blueprint of whiteness. Whiteness in its guise of coloniality describes systems of power and their dynamics that continue to play a significant role in shaping the structures and attitudes within the UK. We think coloniality refers to the often-hidden processes of subjugation that sustain systems and patterns of behaviour that once came from colonialism but now exist as power relations and dynamics shaping how our institutions govern. This is important because the effects of colonialism via coloniality are still being felt by certain groups in society. Grosfoguel (2013) talks about how colonisers committed genocide, "epistemicide" (the killing of knowledge) and the killing of women

---

[2] See Higginbotham (1993).

(femicide—as witches) as the kite mark of colonial barbarity. In Chap. 2, we equated this to the gestation period of whiteness, as we emblemised it by the characterisation of the "savage", as defined by extreme violence. For us, epistemicide, also equates to medicines and modern healthcare being an ill fit for Black people, as it ignores traditional remedies from communities, their contemporary use of which was born out of modern medicines not always generating the best patient experiences for Black people (see Chap. 4 for more details).

Quijano (2007) argues that all power is structured in relations of dominant, exploitation and conflict as social actors compete for control of sex, labour, collective authority and subjectivity/intersubjectivity, their resources and products. However, what is characteristic of global, Eurocentric, capitalist power is that it is organised around two axes that Quijano (2007, p. 168) terms: "the coloniality of power" and "modernity". In terms of our historical identification of whiteness, we would regard Quijano's "modernity" as its birth, when the Negro and its economic function was fully formed (i.e. when it became the site/body in which all mediaeval and early-modern instruments of subjugation were perfected) and "coloniality of power" as the continuation and evolution of whiteness' behavioural patterns. [3] So, in the sense, of "coloniality" describing the ever-present processes of colonial subjugation, we would like to propose, the term "coloniality of whiteness" so as to include the pre-colonial history and ethical origins of whiteness at its conception that still remain with us for example, the concept of the "just war".

As coloniality suggests, there still remains an unequal balance of power between those categorised into distinct minority ethnic groups and those who are racialised as White. "Coloniality of being" (Maldonado-Torres, 2007, p. 242) that focuses on the "lived experiences and not only in the mind" of the colonised has shaped the way in which marginalised African Diaspora people experience health and is an important determinant of their health.

Throughout the COVID-19 pandemic, there has been a notable polarisation of certain populations, including migrants that are disadvantaged by poor, low-paid working conditions and overcrowded living

---

[3] See Chap. 2 for more details.

conditions. Throughout COVID-19, there has also been evidence of how racialisation is shaping the health experience of Black people. This along with other factors such as gender and class has highlighted ongoing systemic structural challenges (Fenton et al., 2020).

Case Example: "Coloniality of Whiteness" in the UK Health System: The "coloniality of whiteness" is illustrated by the current COVID-19 crisis and migrants with No Recourse to Public Funds (NRPF), which is a system that denies access to Public Funds for people with no leave to remain. Migrants that are more likely to be impacted by NRPF are those from developing countries such as the Caribbean and Africa where Consulate arrangements have not been made outside European Economic Area countries. These places are former Colonies of Great Britain and are members of the Commonwealth and are being denied this funding for no good reason. This is an example of "coloniality of whiteness" that is still shaping our institutions and can be described as an extension of colonial violence (Mignolo, 2002; Walter, 2016). During the pandemic we have had evidence of people of colour expected to work in precarious and low-paid roles, losing their jobs and not having the ability to claim from public funds. This has therefore subjected them to find work in areas with greater and more frequent exposure to the COVID-19 virus.

Being Dehumanised by Whiteness

F: About five years ago my mum shared a story about a time when dad worked in the United States for 6 months and left mum with her first child. Although mum had a good network of friends from the church that came to the UK around the same time, most of her friends needed to work so were unavailable to help childmind my brother every time she went to work. Mum retold a story about when she had to go to work and decided to get a childminder, she chose a white lady who she thought would look after my brother at our home. Mum noticed that as the days went by that my brother seemed to become fairly anxious as she came to look after him but thought it was because he was going to miss her.

About two weeks later it became apparent what had been going on. Mum came home to my brother and noted that he had several bruises over him and also that he had been strapped down in the pushchair so tightly that it caused several marks and bruises over his body. My mum was so scared and called the church pastor who was a very good family friend but no one knew how to confront this childminder and ask what happened. When she returned the next day mum did ask (when with the pastor) and she said your "Black Baby" [4] was screaming and I could not shut him up, then she left, mum never saw her again. This was heart breaking and mum talked about the stress this caused, it meant that she could not trust to leave her baby with anyone again and she also had to leave her job.

O: I'm not surprised that this was devastating for your mum to have her child dehumanised and neglected in this way. This thing about not seeing us as human beings deserving of care and protection starts from when we are babies. I can just imagine the hell that Black children left in the care system must go through, where they are not even treated like cherished animals or pets but things to be controlled for the convenience of the so-called care giver.

Your mum's story really resonates at an institutional level for me because this lack of care develops and continues. Your story of neglect and cruelty at your primary school, reminds me of the Child Q case in terms of the lack of care given to a Black girl (see Gamble & McCallum, 2022 but also see The Met, 2022 that shows that Black boys are strip searched in much higher numbers than Black girls). In both cases you and Child Q were adultified, which meant that both of you didn't need the care of adults around you because somehow your race meant that you didn't have an innocence or vulnerability (as a child) to protect. But your baby brother although not adultified was also treated without due care because of his race, somehow being made to suffer from the child minder's lack of ability to see him as a human baby needing care all because of this colour.

F: The other thing mum spoke about was how this experience left her help-less, she did not have confidence or the know how to confront this white woman who felt it was ok to talk to her in that way and most importantly as she described "her Black baby". Mum said that this was a real problem for new people to the country in that people did not mix with those that could help them understand how to challenge people and use services, they had no networks outside of their own communities. People were left to cope without the support from the services.

---

[4] See Chap. 2 to understand the underlying moral degeneracy in this phrase, within the stated context!

The fact that mum could not work meant that she was home and accessible for other friends to go around and socialise. Growing up I had observed women around me functioning as sole breadwinners; single parents juggling two or more low paid jobs; being carers for their immediate and extended family. In addition to all this, I watched people trying to maintain contact and support their wider communities largely through the church to gain some sense of belonging.

Commentary

Your 'Black Baby' [5] was screaming and I could not shut him up.

In Chap. 2, we described at great length how whiteness is a *historical pattern of behaviour* (Clennon, 2019). And that via its religiopolitical incarnation was first distorted into an unethical (i.e. contra to Aristotelian "natural law" [Aristotle, 1944]) societal organisation tool that first sought to strip peoples of their distinguishing and humanising characteristics by homogenising them into one "artificial" grouping (e.g. Saracens) and essentialising them before applying sweeping negative stereotypes to this grouping. We then traced the gestation of whiteness where it used violence to construct its "savage" subjects (e.g. Indigenous of the Americas), where at the same time it sought to diminish human status by conceiving of the "raza" (race) construct of animal pedigree (but applied to humans), as a way of constructing an identification of bloodline (reserved for Jews in living in Spain at the time). Here, we can see how conception grew into gestation by observing the homogenising (and essentialising) of varied groups of peoples using *language* morphing into the pseudo-scientific process of homogenising varied groups of peoples using their "raza" or *bloodlines*. All of this served to gradually strip human beings of their humanity, as we discussed, in ways that would have been alien to the Ancient world, especially when viewed through the Aristotelian "natural law" that was devised for "mankind as a whole" (Aristotle, 1944, pp. [1254b] [1] lines 11–13).

---

[5] See Chap. 2 to understand the underlying moral degeneracy in this phrase, within the stated context!

So, by the time the African body came to embody all of those traits from conception to gestation, whiteness was born in its mature form as the Negro. [6] The African body bore the brunt of whiteness' Saracens, Indigenous and Antisemitic tactics of dehumanisation over the centuries. So, as Robinson (1983) writes, the Negro (the dehumanised African person) [7] was a European fabrication designed to justify the demand for industrial-scale labour by creating a non-human supply to satisfy such a demand. The act of dehumanisation itself and the reason for it, being unethical and morally degenerate, in equal measure.

So, the "Black Baby" of Faye's recollections and the case of Child Q and others undoubtedly emblemise the full legacy of whiteness and its unethical tactic of dehumanisation (i.e. underserving of human care) that has been previously discussed.

Intersectionality: Reasserting Race and Gender?

F: Well for me, school was a very stressful place to be, I had panic attacks about going into school. I remember when we moved house and had to walk for about 15 minutes to get to school (previous house was literally a stone throw across the school road with the lollipop woman), I would walk with my sister and my older brother would always walk ahead. There were a good handful and more occasions when we would meet another two Black boys walking in the same direction. We would wear our school uniforms, but mum would always plait our hair and these boys would laugh at us and called us the N word, [8] telling us how ugly our hair was and calling us blackie.

---

[6] In effect, whiteness was perfected in the disembodied (in the sense of a body with no history or culture) Negro, where there is a Master/Slave Hegelian dialectic (Hegel, 1977) that brings Aristotle's Master/Slave relationship into a dialectical space, which sees the Master as only being validated by the slave whereas the slave finds validation in his work, as described by Clennon (2016). We see whiteness playing out this role of master in this dialectic, as its literal performance can be seen in an imperial context. So, if we regard the Negro merely as a "white man's artifact" (Fanon, 1986 [1952], p. 6), the Negro can be seen as just whiteness in black face and transposed to a market context; "Blackness" (Clennon, 2016).

[7] And later "Black" via market transformation, see Clennon (2016, 2018).

[8] See Chap. 2 and its tracking of the development of whiteness to see why this term is just so heavily loaded. Also see commentary for "Black Baby".

I will never forget how awful those occasions were and to then be subject to a life of misery in school when I knew some of what my parents and friends would warn me to do was to work hard. I really did not want to be there!

O: Faye, this is so sad that these Black boys called you that. I suppose they were also a small visible minority within their school and were parroting the behaviour they saw around them? I can only hope, by now, they have grown out of their internalised hatred of Black women. This is a sad, sad thing but it is also very serious ....

I think that I can only remember being called a Black B [9] once by a white boy at school, one summer's day on the school's tennis courts, which always makes me smile because although I love watching tennis, I still can't play it very well, to this day. But I am fortunate in a way that I didn't experience a huge amount of verbal abuse because my torment mainly came from the school as an institution. My school became infamous for the racist and fatal stabbing of a South Asian boy in the late eighties and this was not some horrendous lone-wolf outlier, it was due to the racist ethos of the school at that time, which didn't know how to treat ethnic minorities, even though we were sizeable and despite having an antiracist policy. But one of my friends who was of Pakistani heritage did regularly get picked on with verbal and physical abuse. He was the first person of my age who showed me what it meant to stand up for yourself, your heritage and who you are. He never ever let anyone shame him or intimidate him either in the playground or on the streets on the way home. He always stood his ground.

F: As the junior school years through to secondary school went by, I had my set of Black and Asian friends but unfortunately, those friends went to a different secondary school and then I began to mix with more white children. I distinctly remember again being in a class in secondary school, hair still plaited and looking quite timid when I was confronted by a group of Black boys again who came to compliment my white, blonde friend and totally disregarded me as unattractive, I soon learnt, it was better not to hang around white blonde girls (or any white girls for that matter) as I would always be overlooked by both Black and white boys.

O: Uh huh … this is where the perception comes from in terms of Black men (in this case, boys) sharing in a patriarchal status that denigrates Black women. Lots to unpack with this one! [10]

---

[9] See Chap. 2 and its tracking of the development of whiteness to see why this term is just so heavily loaded. Also see commentary for "Black Baby".

[10] See Commentary for *Can Intersectionality Work for the Black Male?* section when discussing the limits of Intersectionality when applied to Black men.

F: Yes, but teachers remained dismissive, labelling me as a child that was only good for running, you bet, every sports day I was being selected, I was never encouraged to become academic or learn a musical instrument (despite mum pushing the piano and violin) and hence I left school with very few qualifications … I gave up.

O: I think this would have happened to me also, if I didn't have this strong clique of competitive friends to fire me up and drive me to achieve. My teachers also weren't interested in my academic success but although I was (very) low-key athletic at school, as I was a sprinter and for some random reason was good at shot put, I was an even better musician, so my time was spent playing in the school orchestras. So, my sports teachers never had the opportunity to get their hands on me. Looking back on it, music and my aptitude for it, really saved me in those dark, dark days.

F: Well, I wasn't so lucky, I was seen as strong and not needing support. I remember just before leaving primary school and scared by having my first ever period, I went to tell the teacher as I did not know what to do, she shewed me away and told me to go to the toilet and get some tissues and that was it. In those days, tissue paper was like tracing paper and that was a real problem.

Commentary

Well, I wasn't so lucky, I was seen as strong and not needing support

Black Women, Empire and Intersectionality

Gendered Dehumanisation

Our following discussions about Empire and gender very much pick up where Robinson left off, as regards the formation of the Negro in Chap. 2. However, before discussing intersectionality, we need to quickly remind ourselves of how imperial whiteness shaped gender and what its impact on Black women was (see the next section for a similar discussion for Black men). In Bederman's (1995) *Manliness and Civilization: A Cultural History of Gender and Race in the U.S., 1880–1917*, she writes savage (that is, nonwhite) races … had not yet evolved pronounced sex-ual—and, to some extent, this was precisely what made them savage. Savage men had never evolved the chivalrous instinct to protect their women and children but in-stead forced their women into exhausting drudgery, culti-vating the fields, tending the fires, carrying heavy burdens. Overworked savage women had never evolved the refined delicacy of civilized women.

The above quote was written from the Victorian perspective that the "savage" represented the lack of civility, restraint and refinement that characterised the ideals of humanity at the time. And these ideals of that time were codified by strict expressions of gender difference. See the next section about Victorian manliness for more details, but note here that "civilised women" were expected to be "protected". You will read in the next section that "protected" from the perspective of "manliness" means becoming an extension of "manliness" by being his property along with the "home". Yet many pre-colonial societies evidently did not conceptu-alise gender at all and sought to treat and identify men and women by social relation rather than bodily difference. Oyěwùmí (1997) explains:

> In the Yoruba world, particularly in pre-nineteenth century, Oyo culture, society was conceived to be inhabited by people in relation to one another. That is, the "physicality" of maleness or femaleness did not have social ante-cedents and therefore did not constitute social categories. Social hierarchy was determined by social relations. As noted earlier, how persons were situ-ated in relationships shifted depending on those involved and the particular situation. The principle that determined social organization was seniority, which was based on chronological age. Yoruba kinship terms did not denote gender, and other nonfamilial social categories were not gender-specific either.

So, both Black women and Black men were deemed savages and as a consequence were not assigned a gender.[11] However, reflecting on this characterisation of civility with its full status of humanity, we can see that whiteness is replaying its treatment of the indigenous peoples of the Americas, in the sense of applying its lens of description to others with-out having any reflexive capability. For example, in Chap. 2, we saw that

---

[11] See the next section for an outline of how gender evolved from being a "one-sex" to "two-sex" theory and its moral implications for creating opposing genders.

Sepúlveda viewed the Amerindians as being savage mainly because of their religious sacrificing, whilst totally ignoring the Spanish's own brutal and bloody version of religious sacrifice (for the protection of the Crown) as enacted by the Spanish Inquisition. Similarly, here, imperial whiteness is unable to see [12] beyond its "feelings" (of preconceived and unfounded ideas of superiority) to recognise a sophisticated social ordering around seniority much relating to its own systems of seniority within its male ranks, which, if unblinded, it would have better recognised it as a sort of class system. This lack of reflexion was identified as early as the fourteenth century Ibn Khaldûn in his *The Muqaddimah*, when he noticed how the inhabitants of Mediaeval Northern Europe did not seem to be aware of their whiteness because they were too busy categorising everyone else. [13]

As outlined in the next section about Black Men and imperial whiteness, Black women were equally Saracenised [14] by the process of being homogenised and essentialised into one ethnic African block that itself was characterised as "female", where the "female" embodied the opposite traits of imperial white manliness—that is, lacking control, led by feelings and so on. This led Black women to being seen as wanton sexualised savages as embodied by the Jezebel trope. It is interesting, that the Black men who were equally Saracenised as wanton sexual savages became (and remain) the rapist—there was no allegorical name given to them. We will discuss the reasons for this in the next section.

But what changed for Black women?

Curry (2017, pp. 56–57) sees this as a seminal moment for change!

---

[12] Oyěwùmí (1997, p. 13) echoes this when she writes

> From a cross-cultural perspective, the more interesting point is the degree to which feminism, despite its radical local stance, exhibits the same ethnocentric and imperialistic characteristics of the Western discourses it sought to subvert. This has placed serious limitations on its applicability outside of the culture that produced it.

This also heavily questions the wider use or efficacy of empiricism as employed by whiteness, as it seems that historically it has been unable to take into account its own biases in its outward-looking enquiries.

[13] See Chap. 2.

[14] See note 30.

The most ironic example is the [white] feminist Rebecca Latimer Felton. She began her political career as an advocate for Black women in the 1880s. She began her antirape activism on behalf of a fifteen-year-old Black girl named Adaline Maddox, who was sentenced to five years of hard labor for stealing fifty cents. Felton found that the treatment of young Black women in the convict lease system was horrifying. They were raped by the white guards, forced to have interracial children, and shackled day and night. By 1897, Felton's anti-rape activism had taken a decidedly anti-Black turn. Instead of recognizing the connection the myth of the Black rapist had to the Jezebel myths affecting Black woman, Felton embraced the criminalization and extra-legal murder of Black males.

Here, Curry is describing whiteness' inability to be reflexive,[15] where over time, Black women being raped by white men was irrationally turned into a promotion of the Black Male Rapist trope. Again, we see whiteness' inability to recognise in itself its own moral degeneracy, in this case, sexual profligacy (via societally established Libertine rites of passage for white men (see the next section for more details)) but transferring its disavowed sexual degeneracy onto its subjects that it *sees*. [16] So by turning a blind eye to what was actually happening (i.e. white men raping Black women), Felton used her "feelings" to exploit the situation of Black women to campaign for the rights of white women. And as in the next section, where we find that the Black man becomes the defining concept

---

[15] At this rate, we will have to call this the "Sepúlveda complex" as it seems to be an important recurring feature of the development and application of whiteness. Also see Chap. 2, where we first introduce this. Also see note 29.

[16] Oyěwùmí (1997, p. 2)

> The reason that the body has so much presence in the West is that the world is primarily perceived by sight. The differentiation of human bodies in terms of sex, skin color, and cranium size is a testament to the powers attributed to "seeing." The gaze is an invitation to differentiate.

Seeing, or the "gaze" has indeed been the main tool of imperial domination of whiteness over the centuries but as already argued, it is a gaze that is not reflexive, a gaze that is unable to see itself and a gaze that transfers what it can't see in itself onto others. What we are really talking about is a white (male) gaze, a "whiteness" that is constantly externalising its psyche by constructing physical representations of its psyche (as transferred on to "others"). In effect, whiteness cannot see "others" for who they really are because it is constantly blinded by images of its disavowed self. And sadly, for the rest of humanity, whiteness has not yet become aware of its (moral) blindness!

for white womanhood in terms of the threat of rape, here we can see how this zeitgeist was initially politicised.

In the next section, we discuss how white female domesticity was seen as an extension of the white man's manliness. However, white women took that expectation of "domesticity" and weaponised it by elevating it to the centre of Empire. Whereas the virility of manliness was essential for conquering foreign lands and expanding imperial borders, it was in the *home*, where all of this was translated into foundational teachings that could shape and rear a nation. So, the Victorian home became the single most important tool of imperial national dissemination that whiteness had at that time. And the *home* was the exclusive domain of the Victorian civilised and "docile woman". So despite being demoted to their "feelings", which many white women found unpalatable, [17] they nevertheless carved out a strong political space of imperial power from what was their domestic realm—and of course they had to be protected from Black rapists (who became their source of power), at all costs.

Curry (2017) questions current orthodoxy that suggests that Victorian Black men placed the same emphasis on the home, as their white counterparts for defining *their* manliness. See the next section for an expansion of this. However, (Curry, 2017, p. 60) asks the fundamental question: "Did Black women *desire* to be placed within the home and call for the protection of Black men?" (italics, original). This is a crucial question to ponder because Newman (1999, p. 20) observes:

> As the personal and political struggles of Anna Julia Cooper, Ida B. Wells, and Mary Church Terrell suggest, civilization, racial progress, and woman's protection within the home were interconnected in ways that made it impossible for [B]lack women to repudiate altogether the prevailing ideologies of the cult of domesticity and true womanhood. Like their white counterparts, [B]lack women reformers also used evolutionist discourses of civilization to justify their own social activism. They asserted their duty to "elevate" and "uplift" the masses of [B]lack women, upholding the values of domesticity, chastity, temperance, and piety that the white middle classes considered to be evidence of a civilized race.

---

[17] See note 21.

It is important to note that it was actually Black women who used *domesticity* as *their* newly-found means for not just achieving (Black) women's rights (as was the want of their white counterparts, who wanted be seen as equals in the imperial project) but for achieving the uplift of the entire Black 'race'. This unfortunately meant that appropriating imperial whiteness became their only way of achieving racial uplift. Higginbotham (1993) provides an excellent account of how white women actively encouraged the development of Black women's female domestic sensitivities, as a means of civilising them so that these Black women could disseminate imperial civility in *their* homes (dominions); the roots of the Politics of Respectability (Higginbotham, 1993). Sadly, modelling imperial domesticity that already had the Black Rapist as its existential blueprint in terms of threat, meant the Black men were left behind in this era of image-reform, as their Black Rapist image remained even in what became the social movement of Black domesticity for racial uplift. However, this irony was not entirely lost on all Black female activists of the time, as notably, Wells-Barnett (2014 [1892], p. 36) writes:

> Humanity abhors the assailant of womanhood, and this charge upon the Negro at once placed him beyond the pale of human sympathy. With such unanimity, earnestness and apparent candor was this charge made and reiterated that the world has accepted the story that the Negro is a monster which the Southern white man has painted him.

Ok. Now we've provided a brief imperial context for gender, as it related to Black women, we can now better understand the fundamental implications of intersectionality, which we will discuss later in the next section.

The Relevance of Intersectionality for Black Women

Intersectionality in our community conversations can on the surface, provide a framework to explore how the underlying systems shape the health experience for Black women. Intersectionality as originally conceptualised by Crenshaw (1991), is broadly understood as the intersecting identities between gender and race for Black women, specifically in

US law where they were protected by neither gender anti-discrimination nor race anti-discrimination laws. This lens can be useful if looking at for example, the colonial killing (and raping) of Black women being mapped across to contemporary poor healthcare of Black women and child birth, where via institutional neglect and dehumanisation, they are five times more likely to die from complications to do with their pregnancy (Knight, 2019). Or that Black women are more likely to be viewed as promiscuous and highly sexualised single mothers with many children (Rosenthal & Lobel, 2016)—the imperial Jezebel trope still making its presence felt. Or that as "savage" beasts, Black women can endure higher (inhuman) levels of pain (Hoffman et al., 2016). Also see Prather et al. (2018), who wrote about Marion J Sims (1813–1883), who is regarded as the 'father of modern gynaecology' because he undertook surgical procedures on Black women after childbirth without available analgesia or consent.

We can see that there are many health-damaging stereotypes that have stemmed from imperial whiteness where Black women had to be socialised by their parents and communities to be 'strong Black women'. [18] And we know that these stereotypical ideologies continue, based on the view that Black people are uncivilised and deserving of being dominated and treated in inhumane ways. But to really see if intersectionality is still a relevant concept, we will actually need to check it against the needs of Black men (whose race and gender also intersect), as we track how imperial whiteness shaped gender for Black men and its persistence to this day.

Intersectionality and the Black Male?

F: Growing up I had observed women around me functioning as sole breadwinners.
O: Yup! I do think we're going to have to explore why these women were often the sole breadwinners and main carers for their children. I think there is definitely something to be said about why the men were unable to

---

[18] See Cole (2018) "The trope of the steely, resolute black woman is ingrained in society, and helps fuel a growing problem with depression and self-harm".

find employment to look after their families, in the first place.[19] There does seem to be a missing part of this story when looking at this issue.

F: That might be true but nevertheless Black women *were* treated as subordinate, we were lesser than others based on our race and gender whether at school, college, university, or in employment. In fact, this lesser treatment where we were viewed as not as good as others, was commonplace.

There were so many social problems in families where older children would end up being imprisoned for criminal offences such as drug dealing and robberies. Many of these Black young men dated and had children with white women. What I noted was that the type of boys that laughed at us going to school were the ones involved in drug gangs and territorial wars, it was very masculine. They were failed by their school and this was their way of displaying power and control.

O: OK, we're getting down to the brass tacks now. Yes, I can see how the subordination of Black women can be viewed through an intersectional lens, where her perception as being "not as good as others" because of her race and gender is a real thing. But if we apply the same intersectional lens, as it stands to try to make sense of Black women being oppressed by everyone else, including Black men (boys in your case), what you are describing appears to be a version of toxic Black Masculinity that is deviant and nurtures hatred of Black women. I think that this is a popular image of a type of Black Masculinity but we're going to have to unpack that in terms of the historical, social and economic factors that places Black men into these precarious positions that start from childhood by failed by their schools, as you observed from your reflections.

---

[19] For example, Collins (1990, p. 61)

The disappearance of well-paid manufacturing jobs for Black working-class men suggests that young African-American women view the dual-income, working-class family as a hoped-for, albeit difficult-to-achieve, option. The alternative open to past generations of Blacks—intact marriages based on reasonably steady, adequately paid jobs for Black men and reliable yet lesser-paid jobs for Black women—is less available in the advanced capitalist welfare state. Black working-class women, especially those employed in the government sector as clerical workers, are more likely to find steady employment. But the income of Black working-class wives cannot compensate for the loss of Black men's incomes. Despite expressing support for dominant "family values" ideology, Black working-class women may find themselves as single mothers.

For me, it is this precariousness (i.e. institutional and societal failure of Black boys) that points to a Black male vulnerability that is the missing link behind this characterisation. I am not sure intersectionality is an adequate framework for understanding the whole picture for Black men. For instance, I can remember in my family that it was the Black men that were constantly being stopped and searched under the then suss laws (not the women!) and it got so bad for them that they emigrated to the US for a better life. Questions around the state's need to criminalise young Black men have to be asked. Why are young Black men disproportionately represented in the criminal justice system? We can't really just say it is because they are inherently deviant as per the stereotype. To leave it at that would be very dangerous, indeed. So, we'll definitely have to bookmark this for the commentary section for now. But make no mistake, this popularised image of the deviant Black male has devastating implications for his health and health seeking behaviours!

Commentary

Toxic Black Masculinity that is deviant (i.e. hypersexual and hyperaggressive)

Empire and the Black Male Gender

The above quote refers to the specificity of male-gendered dehumanisation through the schemata of whiteness. To understand more precisely where this perception comes from, we will need to look at how gender is actually an imperial construct and how the latter is a continuation of the development of whiteness, as discussed in Chap. 2 and in the previous section for Black women.

Tosh (2016, pp. Chap 3, section II, para 3) in his *Manliness and Masculinities in Nineteenth-Century Britain* tells us that the driving force of Empire building in Britain was the masculinity or manliness as embodied by strong, physically able (white) men (from all classes). The imperial man followed Aristotelian natural law where men were superior to women:

This framework has the great advantage of foregrounding the relational aspect of gender: within an insistent metaphor of polarization, masculinity can only be understood in relation to its 'other', and during this period the feminine became a much more pervasive 'other' than the child, the slave or the savage, each of which provided alternative reverse images of man.

The above quote is interesting because Aristotelian natural law held women and slaves (both subordinates of the master of the house) as having distinctly different natures but playing *equally* important roles in the Ancient Greek household (unlike in Victorian imperial Britain).[20, 21] In this imperial incarnation, however, women become an oppositional

---

[20] Aristotle (1944, p. [1252a] [1] lines 21–28)

> The first coupling together of persons then to which necessity gives rise is that between those who are unable to exist without one another for instance the union of female and male for the continuance of the species (and this not of deliberate purpose, but with man as with the other animals and with plants there is a natural instinct to desire to leave behind one another being of the same sort as oneself); and the union of natural ruler and natural subject for the sake of security (for he that can foresee with his mind is naturally ruler and naturally master, and he that can do these things with his body is subject and naturally a slave; so that master and slave have the same interest).

[21] However, Wollstonecraft (2002 [1792], p. 81) complains that women were demoted to the level of "feelings", alluding to the Aristotelain "tamed beast":

> Ignorance is a frail base for virtue! Yet, that it is the condition for which woman was organized, has been insisted upon by the writers who have most vehemently argued in favour of the superiority of man; a superiority not in degree, but essence; though, to soften the argument, they have laboured to prove, with chivalrous generosity, that the sexes ought not to be compared; man was made to reason, woman to feel: and that together, flesh and spirit, they make the most perfect whole, by blending happily reason and sensibility into one character.

"other" that in disavowed form, defines masculinity, [22] whilst the child, slave and the savage act as clear examples of what men are *not*.

Here, we can see that whiteness in its imperial form is primarily gendered male in order to project national power in overseas colonies. But to be considered fully "masculine", he needed a household consisting of a wife and children (i.e. underlying implication of the need to assert sexual control over the wife). However, in terms of sexual control over women, Tosh (2016, pp. Chap 3, section I, para 8) continues:

> My second instance of enduring masculinity is the sexual rite of passage of young men on the threshold of manhood. In terms of peer-group standing this was no less a badge of masculine status than the household headship which was meant to follow a few years later. In the mid-eighteenth century it would seem that sowing wild oats was often commended not only by a well-born young man's companions, but by his parents also.

This sexual freedom unofficially afforded to young men was often referred to as Libertine. However, for this sexuality to be nurtured into a commonly accepted phase of growing up, it had to be supported by homosocial structures. Tosh (2016, pp. Chap. 3, section II, para 5) explains these structures as:

> the somewhat infelicitous neologism 'homosociality'. ('Fraternalism' is an older and more attractive term, but it is best reserved for more institution-

---

[22] Laqueur (1990) traces how from Classical times the female body (reproductive system) was seen as an inversion of the male body (reproductive system) by correlating ovaries to testes, and so on. So, although women were seen as inferior to men as the male version of reproductive organs had primacy over the female "inversion" both men and women were seen as "one sex". However, post Enlightenment, Laqueur traces how the "two sex" theory became popular, where men's and women's bodies were seen as not inversions of each other but as two distinct opposing forms where the formally correlated parts of the reproductive system were regarded as antithetical opposites. Antithesis was important here because with it, certain opposing characteristics were ascribed to female and male bodies. Tosh (2016, pp. Chap. 3, Section II, para 2):

> With the two-sex model came an increasingly dichotomized notion of mind and temperament. For men, this meant an intensified emphasis on rationality as against emotionality, energy rather than repose, constancy instead of variability, action instead of passivity, and taciturnity rather than talkativeness.

alized forms of male association based on an ideology of brotherhood.) Passing time with male companions was the traditional leisure occupation of men at all levels of society, whether in the informal conviviality of an alehouse or in more elaborate craft associations and fraternities. This reflected the central role of peer approval in confirming masculine status, as well as the need for support networks for men who were seeking to survive and prosper in business or employment.

Ok. So far, we have seen how imperial whiteness is primarily gendered as male with an oppositional and life giving (in terms of masculine identity) female gender characterised by docility (in distinct opposition to male virility amongst other oppositional qualities). We can see that (male) whiteness is founded on the sexual domination of women (i.e. a wife) in the household (which itself is a visible marker of manliness) and the Libertine sexual freedom thought necessary to eventually grow into the epitome of mature self-controlled manliness (as depicted by the household and important validating homosocial (patriarchal) networks). [23] Finally, also remembering that the child, slave and the savage acted as profound examples of what (manly) white men were definitely *not*! So, what has all of this got to do with the Black Masculinity? Curry (2017, p. 42) in his *Man Not* writes from a US context that:

> it was the newly won freedom of Black men that launched the theorization of our modern concept of gender. Their freedom inspired ethnologists and feminists to give accounts of femininity that were vulnerable to male violence. It was ultimately the threat of Black male citizenship that gave substance to our current concept of gender in whites. Under nineteenth-century ethnological schemes, Black men and women were of a different evolutionary stock of beings. Gender did not exist because of their Blackness.

---

[23] These networks that create the norms of Victorian (male) power very much speak to Bourdieu's (1977) theory of "habitus" or field (like a club) that creates a common world view for its members. This world view is what holds the club together and the club has the power to determine its own terms of reference whenever it wants and for however long it wants (Bourdieu calls this a "taste-making" power)—a network of power that governs its specific part of society (think of the fields of the judiciary, law enforcement, education, etc.). These social networks could be well viewed as Victorian patriarchy, especially as they influenced the professional fields of the day.

Indeed, we already know from Tosh (2016) that as savages or slaves, Black men were examples of what white men or manliness were not. Black men were constantly held as the opposite of white men, who were the epitome of masculinity. [24] We also know that white masculinity upheld the household and the accompanying wife as a marker for its manliness, which means that the wife and her virtue had to be protected at all costs. So, we know that Black men could not be seen as "masculine" so as to upset the then dominant idea of (white) masculinity also meaning that membership of any homosocial networks enjoyed by white manliness would also have been impossible.

We can see that one of the historical hallmarks of whiteness from Chap. 2, at play is this slave/savage characterisation of the Negro. Remember as its goal, it has its unethical drive towards dehumanising its subject (i.e. Saracens being homogenised, essentialised and collectively demonised, Sepúlveda and the indigenous "savage" peoples and the "raza" referring to Jewish heritage). Hegel (1991, pp. 110–111) in his 1822–1830 work, *The Philosophy of History*:

> In Negro life the characteristic point is the fact that conscious-ness has not yet attained to the realization of any substantial objective existence—as, for example, God, or Law—in which the interest of man's volition is involved and in which he realizes his own being. This distinction between himself as an individual and the universality of his essential being, the African in the uniform, undeveloped oneness of his existence has not yet attained; so that the Knowledge of an absolute Being, an Other and a Higher than his individual self, is entirely wanting. The Negro, as already observed, exhibits the natural man in his completely wild and untamed state.

The above quote from Hegel rather seals the fate of whiteness as an unethical form of moral degeneracy that explicitly dehumanises the African to the level of a "untamed" beast driven by its "feelings" or in Hegel's case, by its sense of "self". See Chap. 4 to read how wrong Hegel was about the "Negro" and "God", in so doing, perfectly illustrating the

---

[24] Using Fanon and Lacan as conceptual frameworks to help understand the pathology and drive of (male-gendered) whiteness, see Clennon (2016) for a psychoanalytical explanation of this "negative" role that was, of course, disavowed.

Sepúlveda complex. However, Hegel's intellectual sleight of hand is to replace Aristotelian "reason" with Victorian Christianity as the marker for humanity, much like how Sepúlveda used Spanish Catholicism to the same ends in the Americas.

Curry (2017) observes that the non-human status of the Negro of the eighteenth century did in fact develop into a nineteenth-century admission of the Negro into humanity but only as a lower class of human. [25] In fact, the Negro in this quasi-human form was held in a perpetual state of childlikeness, where slavery was its only hope of redemption or betterment (that obviously would never come). So, if we go back to imperial manliness, 'the wife' was an "other" to the master of house in a way that defined his masculinity as oppositional to her femininity (e.g. his being virile against her being docile, his being taciturn against her being talkative and emotional, etc.). As already mentioned, if we see 'the wife' as a marker for masculinity that as an extension of the man has to be protected, we can see that the Black man also performed the pervasive 'other' for the white woman, 'the wife'. Curry argues that the biological maleness of the Black man could not confer patriarchal [26] alliance but only an existential threat to imperial masculinity via an ever-existing threat to the white woman, 'the wife'. So, imperial femininity became defined by fear of rape (loss of virtue and by extension manliness of the husband).

However, to justify the threat posed by this child-like Black man who is a 'Man-Not' (see Curry's [2017] book title) his lack of gender assignment had to be accounted for, somehow. How they did that, was to ascribe a gender to the African continent and its people. In an extremely

---

[25] An evolution of whiteness?

[26] Interestingly, Paul (2009) writes about this in his exploration of the slave autobiography of Olaudah Equiano called *The Interesting Narrative of the Life of Olaudah Equiano, or Gustavus Vassa, the African, Written by Himself* (Equiano, 2005 [1789]), where he uses Fanon's (1986 [1952]) *Black Skin, White Masks* as a psychological entry point into understanding what must have been racial contradictions within Equiano in his psyche, who in one of his vignettes describes how he painted his own face white as a disguise. Despite Equiano's efforts to code switch (Ogbu, 2004), he still found (rather obviously from our vantage point) that his race and gender always made him vulnerable to recapture and no matter his strides in education or business, his personal agency was always contingent on the pragmatism (and mercy) of whiteness … to his detriment.

Saracen-esque move, Africa was gendered female[27, 28] because of its pre-
ponderance of female rulers and sophisticated governing systems. But
like Sepúlveda, they ignored what they saw and instead, in a similar process to Saracenisation, imposed their imperial sense of (white) femininity,
[29] onto a whole continent and its people! This meant that the Black child-
like non-man (Man-Not) was also feminised as lacking in self-control
and being emotionally led.[30] What this meant was that Black men had to
be *inherently* prone to abusing their masculinities due to their child-like
and *feminine* un-tempered natures. This attribution of sexual deviancy
given to the Man-Not is especially pernicious as it would seem to come
from an unacknowledged fear generated by *their* own Libertine attitudes
towards (white) male rite of passage sexual practices. This, ultimately
meant that Man-Nots had to be a *natural* threat to imperial femininity

---

[27] See Michelet (1867, p. 133)

"Africa; is a woman; her races are feminine," says, very truly, Gustavus d'Eichthall. The rev-
elation of Africa; in the red race of Egypt was in the reign of the great Isis (Osiris was secondary). In many of the black tribes of Central Africa, the women rule; and they are as intelligent
as they are amiable and kind. We see this in Hayti, where they not only improvise charming
little songs for their festivals, inspired by their affections, but in business operations solve
very complicated mental problems.   .

Also see Hunt (1863, p. 16) "There is no doubt that the Negro brain bears a great re-semblance
to a European female or child's brain" and Dunn (1866, p. 13) "He manifests a propensity for
pleasure, music, dancing, physical enjoyments, and conversation, while his inconstancy of impres-
sions and of all the feelings are those of a child".

[28] What were the pre-colonial social relationships that were being observed and so severely misun-
derstood by European explorers? See Oyěwùmí (1997) for more details about African "genders".
Also see Chap. 4 for details of pre-colonial understandings of social, health and community
epistemologies.

[29] Which remember was rendered the complete negative opposite of manliness, so it was emotional
and lacking in self-control and moderation.

[30] See note 21 where Wollstonecraft (2002 [1792]) bemoaned the patriarchal tendency to reduce
women to their "feelings". Where this becomes "peak" whiteness is that like Sepúlveda who ignored
the violence of his own Spanish Inquisition to condemn the indigenous people's violent rituals,
similarly, imperial whiteness ignored its own unofficially societally sanctioned Libertine life style of
sexual excess and abandon as part of its masculine rites of passage, yet judged the people they colonised for what they understood of their sexual practices. Transference or superimposition appears
to be a strong pattern of behaviour for whiteness, where it projects its own unacknowledged (disavowed) demons onto the peoples it encounters. And as this process is disavowed it becomes virtu-
ally impossible for whiteness to face itself and mature. This perhaps explains how the Black male
body becomes fetishsised, feminised and made vulnerable under the white male gaze (whiteness).
Also see note 16.

(white women and by extension white men and their manliness) and in turn, had to be severely punished. [31]

We can see that our underlying societal beliefs about a deviant Black Masculinity are actually a social construct of historical whiteness that emerged from imperial gender theories (i.e. Laqueur, 1990 and "two-sex"). Curry (2017) argues that not only could Black men not join existing (white) patriarchal (homosocial) networks but because of their *severe* punishment for being Man-Nots they were unable to form their own patriarchal networks due to their severe lack of social and economic resources. Rose (1982, p. 29) fills this out with detailed historical accounts of life on nineteenth-century Southern plantations (the blueprint for post slavery economics for Black women and men) with her chapter, "The Domestication of Domestic Slavery":

> To make the "domestic institution" still more complicated, while the plantation community was a patriarchy and the planter's family a matriarchy, the domesticity in the enslaved cabin at the quarters was, ironically, about as close an approximation to equality of the sexes as the nineteenth century provided. An androgynous world was born, weirdly enough, not of freedom, but bondage.

Rose makes clear that the slave owner, his (sometimes, her) family and their slaves were subsumed into a Christian framework of looking after a household, where the moral virtue of the slaveowner was epitomised by his public kindness to his "people" (slaves). In practice, this meant that

---

[31] Whether physically in terms of castration (in extreme cases) or societally, in terms of economic "castration", especially today via lower educational opportunities (higher numbers of temporary and permanent exclusions), as well as lower employment outcomes, higher numbers of police harassment (e.g. see The Met, 2022 for data on strip searches), higher numbers of incarceration, higher numbers in mental health institutions. The list goes on. The recent killing of George Floyd is a historical but also a regular occurrence that can be traced back to colonialism and the lynching of Black men during the Jim Crow era in the US (Jones, 2005). George Floyd sparked a heightened resurgence of the Black Lives Matter movement where the brutal killing shone a light globally on the mistreatment of Black people across the world (Garza, 2020). These racial micro-aggressions, discrimination and disregard for the Black male body impacts upon the overall health of Black men subjecting them to higher rates of mental ill-health and overall poor health (Jones, 2005). The prevalence and de-prioritisation of targeted prostate cancer treatment, harsher treatment in the mental health system with drugs and not talking therapies and the lack of targeted HIV treatment in African Diaspora communities are all examples of de-prioritised care. For acute de-prioritisation, also see Long (2022) who reports how UK paramedics failed to treat a Black Man under arrest for epileptic seizures because they thought he was pretending, despite his having a medical history of epilepsy.

the slave owner was the patriarch of the plantation and his slaves, whilst his wife was the de facto matriarch of the family, looking after the domestic running of the house. This idea of domesticity reflects Tosh's analysis of nineteenth-century masculinity in Britain at that time, [32] which we are sure was replicated in British slave plantations of the time. But the main point Rose illustrates is that the un-gendered nature of the slaves who were seen as beasts of burden meant that there were, in fact, no imitations of patriarchy within *their* households.

The reason for outlining the origins of the toxic Black Masculinity trope to this extent is that its creation in imperial whiteness continues to exert a "coloniality of power" (see Mignolo, 2000, 2002; Mignolo & Escobar, 2010) or as we would call it a "coloniality of whiteness" over the ways in which institutions (and in our case the health market) continue treat Black Men, as undeserving of care but deserving of punishment (because of sexual profligacy, hyperviolence, etc.) in order to contain an imaginary threat to now contemporary whiteness.

Black Male Health and Imperial Whiteness

O: How did you see this manifesting in the health of the Black men you grew up with?

F: As I look back, I do note the health of our Black men and their disengagement from services. The day that one of the church elders who didn't manage his diabetes had his leg amputated frightened me and he spoke about how he didn't know how to manage his diabetes. In my conversations with community members, men would talk about how difficult it was to engage with health professionals because they did not understand their Jamaican language/accent.

O: Ok. I think that the reasons for Black Men to disengage from health services, very much has a lot to do with how they are characterised more widely. What I mean here, is that their perceived lack of humanity is manifested in an institutional neglect that you hinted at with your brother and

---

[32] Where despite being head of the household, too much time spent at home could often cause conflict with his wife, if he interfered with the wife's domestic control of the house.

that institutional neglect is informed by the toxic image of violent Black masculinity now replaced by excuses around accents and their intelligibility that you touched upon earlier. [33]

One of our community partners added:

I cannot say them [other men] and not refer to myself in this, there are some things that I will just not do despite what they [health professional] advise. That test that you have for prostate cancer, I will not let anyone near me, yes its pride but … and I know that as a Black man I could be at higher risk of getting the cancer.

Commentary

Post Traumatic Slave Syndrome

It is clear that the Black Male body via its (past physical) punishments for being male, [34] has undergone traumatic abuse historically and it is equally interesting that our male community member seems to be frozen into a type of Black Masculinity that he refers to as "pride", which sees him associate a rectal examination for prostate cancer as shameful or even harmful. To explain this phenomenon, DeGruy Leary's (2005) *Post traumatic slave syndrome: America's legacy of enduring injury and healing* argues that the form of oppression experienced by Black people during slavery and contemporary institutional racism (markers of the *historical patterns of behaviour* from whiteness) can result in collective multigenerational trauma and grief that can be directly or indirectly experienced by Black people. These chronic stressors can influence the individual over the life course and this can impact greatly upon their physical, intellectual and emotional development.

---

[33] See Balibar (1991) who writes about how discussions around race have over time been morphed into discussions about culture that are still underpinned by racist and racial ideologies. So, conversations around the intelligibility of African Diaspora accents can very much be seen as an extension of the "savage" and civility codes of whiteness that have been discussed in this chapter, especially as it relates to Black men.

[34] See note 31.

The inheritability of Post Traumatic Slave Syndrome can also be described by epigenetics, where the expression of genes is altered without changes to the actual DNA code and where this expression can be modified according to the conditions in which we live. The role of genetic factors and the role they play in health disparities have been debated by scientists, however, race by itself (i.e. minus psychosocial factors) is a poor proxy for genetic background, meaning that genetics, cannot account for the racial disparities in health (Braun, 2002, 2006; Williams et al., 2019; Payne-Sturges et al., 2021). However, there is evidence (e.g. see Ammous et al., 2021; Evans-Campbell, 2008; Bombay et al., 2014; Graff, 2014; Shackel, 2018) suggesting that the effects of trauma, which includes events such as colonisation, slavery and continued systemic discrimination (i.e. psychosocial factors), seem to be epigenetically transmitted (inherited) and then manifested as accelerated ageing with its concomitant effects of ill-health such as cardiovascular disease (i.e. weathering, see Chap. 2), although Kim et al. (2022) did find that healthy eating can mitigate some of the epigenetic effects of weathering (thank goodness!).

We know that Black men experience poor health treatment due to the negative racist attitudes (the roots of which we have just outlined), regarding their physical characteristics or abilities. For example, NICE decisions that fail to meet the QALY's [35] cost-effectiveness threshold include a new drug called "abiraterone" to treat prostate cancer that has not been approved, despite evidence of an increase in the health and life expectancy of individuals with prostate cancer. There is historical evidence to indicate that Black men have a higher risk of prostate cancer compared to White men and other ethnic groups (Odedina et al., 2009). Several pieces of literature (e.g. Rebbeck et al., 2013; McGinley et al., 2016) support this and provide evidence that globally, Caribbean and African men are three times more likely to be diagnosed with aggressive prostate cancer than White men in the UK and develop it at least five years earlier. So, it would appear that Caribbean and African men who need abiraterone the most are being deprived of an increase in health and life expectancy, seemingly for the hidden reasons or attitudes (i.e. QALYfying "the value

---

[35] See Chap. 2 for more details about the Quality Adjusted Life Years (QALYs) and National Institute of Care Excellence (NICE).

of [their] lives to be below the desirable level of well-being), that have already been suggested in this chapter. [36]

Does Intersectionality really work as fair concept for theorising both Black female and Black male genders?

So, having looked at gender from the perspective of imperial whiteness, Lugones' (2008) concept of the "coloniality of gender" makes sense to us, as we can see the persistence of these imperial ideas of gender at play today in the running of our institutions. However, we disagree with the implicit notion that gender (only) refers to "women" and their societal role because, as we have discussed, this blind spot (limited definition) can have catastrophic implications for Black men and *their* gender. This omission is so serious that Curry (2017, p. 7) writes "[f]or Sylvia Wynter, genre indicates the disruption of the order founded on European man and woman, which is expressed by the term of gender".

It is this very point about gender that for us puts intersectionality on very shaky grounds, especially since we are equally concerned about Black male health. Intersectionality fails to provide a clear enough framework to help explain the social factors and their history behind lower health outcomes for Black men. We think that the reason for this is that intersectionality has unwittingly used imperial whiteness as its foundation. In

---

[36] Also see Jones (1981 [1993]) who writes about the Tuskegee Study where Black men were denied effective treatment for syphilis so that the United States Public Health Service could carry out experiments to understand the natural progression of the disease. In reviewing the book, Geiger (1981) concludes:

And there lies the central contribution of "Bad Blood," for Mr. Jones, who was a Kennedy fellow in bioethics at Harvard University and a senior research fellow at the Kennedy Institute of Ethics at Georgetown University, has gone back to the beginning and demonstrated that the study was not an aberration. He has searched the archives, reviewed the medical reports, read the physicians' official letters (full of references to "ignorant darkies" and "the Ethiopian population"). The Tuskegee Study, he shows, had its roots in the Social Darwinism and pseudoscientific racial beliefs that infected American medicine—and much of American life and society—through most of the 19th and early 20th centuries, with endless warnings of a "syphilis-soaked race," and of an inferior people with large genitalia and small brains being destroyed by freedom.

Also see Brooks (2022, para 1) who reports on an apology issued on behalf of The City of Philadelphia "for the unethical medical experiments performed on mostly Black inmates at its Holmesburg Prison from the 1950s through the 1970s."

his *Decolonising the Intersection*, Curry (2021) examines how Kimberlé Crenshaw based her conception of (Black female) gender on an earlier *Dominance Theory* conceived by MacKinnon (1989, pp. Chap. 9, para 1)

> If sexuality is central to women's definition and forced sex is central to sexuality, rape is indigenous, not exceptional, to women's social condition. In feminist analysis, a rape is not an isolated event or moral transgression or individual interchange gone wrong but an act of terrorism and torture within a systemic context of group subjection, like lynching.

In the context of the gender formation by (and within) imperial whiteness, defining women in relation to rape is a direct legacy of gendered female whiteness. Remember, imperial white women were subject to the control of their white "manly" husbands and with this control came protection. And with protection this enabled white women to build imperial *homes* from which they could rear the nation and Empire. So, we need to keep in mind that it was this *domestic* status that enabled early (white) women's rights advocates to demand a seat at the imperial table with the men. But we also need to be mindful of what these (white) women needed protection from. It was the Black Male Rapist. The threat of rape was the instrument that defined and promoted their domestic womanhood as needing to be *protected*. And as we have discussed, this need for protection was an imperial civility code that white women's rights advocates even wanted to impose on Black women at that time for the purposes of racial uplift.

So, to equate the ever-present *fear* of rape by the Black Male Rapist (who gave them their "protected" status) with the ever-present *reality* of lynching, which was a special instrument reserved for both Black women and especially Black men in terms of removing the threat of rape via physical castration, seems distasteful to say the very least! Even if we concede that the spectre of the Black Male Rapist (of white women) had receded by that time (Griffin, 1971), its symbolic power and "threat" would still inform ongoing debates about rape. [37]

---

[37] See note 40 for a brief expansion on inter and intra-rape theory.

We can also see that grouping all (white) women's sexuality into this category/definition of "forced sex" is of course an older mechanism of whiteness, namely, Saracenisation, only where in this context, the homogenised and essentialised group is attributed values of virtue and purity (which must be protected).

Curry (2021) continues to explain that Crenshaw also sought to apply this definition to Black womanhood because she believed that Black women were also oppressed as women in a patriarchal system. This has surprising parallels with imperial Black women assuming the same values as their white counterparts in elevating the home but in their case for racial uplift. In both instances, in order to develop their strategies for power (sharing) there had to be a need for the Black Male Rapist to maintain the threat. As Curry shows, there was (and is) no substantial evidence for Crenshaw to have built her beliefs on the predatory Black Male Rapist trope even though it was a fashionable doctrine of gender theorisation in the 1970s and 1980s. [38] So rather than interrogate the effects of patriarchy on Black women that came from imperial white manliness, regarding Black women as wanton savage Jezebels onto which they could project their Libertine fantasies with impunity (dehumanising them as sexually disposable, as reported by Rebecca Latimer Felton in the 1880s), Crenshaw chose to blame Black women's oppression on Black men by maintaining the Black Male Rapist trope. [39] This is even more egregious because Crenshaw seems to forget the existential control patriarchy had

---

[38] See note 40.

[39] This is of course, complex because intra-rape rates are high, see note 40 but not for the essentialist pathological reasons put forth by what was formally imperial whiteness, now existing as a "coloniality of gender" (Lugones, 2008) or "coloniality of whiteness".

(has) on Black masculinity via not just the threat of but the actual continual lynching of Black men. [40]

The hidden influences of imperial whiteness and gender formation also continue to be felt in the influential work of hooks (2004), where Curry (2021) explains that hooks theorises how the patriarchal existential control of Black masculinity can be viewed as manifesting in (over)compensatory behaviours of Black men. So, hooks in her way also amplifies the Black Male Rapist trope because as Curry shows, hooks' theorising comes from a pathological position that this sexual violence is not caused by external factors, as we have discussed in terms of patriarchy but is *inherent* to the Black male.

---

[40] Curry (2021) gives a good account of the centrality of "rape" and the Black man to US sociological studies in the 1970s and 1980s from Amir's (1971) work that showed that white women were not in danger of being raped by Black men but Black women were (bearing in mind his study took place in major urban areas in Philadelphia, where there are higher numbers of large Black communities) to Curtis' (1976) work that used the "intra-racial" theory of rape to pathologise Black men. Amir disproved the "inter-racial" theory of rape that placed white women at risk. Amir demonstrated the "intra-racial" theory of rape that applied to rape within Black communities (which also implied that white men were predominantly responsible for raping white women in predominantly white communities). Amir put this phenomenon down to subcultural reasons derived from socioeconomic factors in his Philadelphia study. However, Curtis (1975) took these findings and interpreted them as a pathological component of Black male sexuality. What is important to note here is that the Sepúlveda complex of whiteness, as described earlier, makes yet another appearance because when Griffin (1971, p. 35) wrote:

> [t]he same men and power structure who victimise women are engaged in raping Vietnam, raping Black people and the very earth we live upon .... As the symbolic expression of white male hierarchy, rape is the quintessential act of our civilisation

Curtis took exception to this statement by emphasising the high rates of intra-rape in Black communities, whilst acknowledging that inter-rape rates were low but resolutely remaining totally unable to acknowledge the high rates of intra-rape in white communities, which Griffin was pointing out in her work. However, the moral blindness of whiteness of not being able to see itself is turned into moral degeneracy when Curtis (1976) finally does admit that rape is indeed an instrument of white patriarchy but Black men have adopted it with greater savagery because of (wait for it … Saracenisation-alert!) their pathological preoccupation with their phalluses. However, as previously discussed, what we are really discussing is the disavowed Libertine abandon and moral degeneracy of whiteness that is projected onto the Black man, as whiteness desperately needs to cast him (i.e. fix in place) as the Rapist for its very existence!

Conclusion

The reason why we assert that Intersectionality is a weak analytical framework for understanding the gender formations and relations between Black women and Black men is that it robs Black men of any theoretical agency to define themselves for themselves. This is why tracing whiteness as a historical pattern of behaviour over the longue durée has been so important for us because it has allowed us to see its influence and impact on, what would first appear to be a Black liberatory gender theory. We also think that such a perspective on whiteness can allow us to see continuities in its application to Public Health.

In the next chapter we will take a break from our decolonial enquiries into the "coloniality of whiteness" and take an approach characterised by decolonisation (Mignolo, 2002) and the ethnophilosophy of Ubuntu (see Oruka, 1990; Sefa Dei, 2014; Mbiti, 1970) where we will use our community partners' thoughts about health and health management as clues to finding past (traditional) African health traditions. We will attempt to excavate their "traditional heritage knowledges" (Clennon, 2022) to see if we can get a glimpse of pre-colonial health epistemologies that exist as remnants in today's African Diaspora and whether any of them can be updated and reimagined for the twenty-first century (via Ubuntu's critical philosophy see, Gyekye, 1995).

Works Cited

Amir, M. (1971). *Patterns in Forcible Rape*. University of Chicago Press.
Ammous, F., Zhao, W., Ratliff, S. M., Mosley, T. H., Bielak, L. F., Zhou, X., et al. (2021). Epigenetic Age Acceleration Is Associated with Cardiometabolic Risk Factors and Clinical Cardiovascular Disease Risk Scores in African Americans. *Clinical Epigenetics, 13*, 55. https://doi.org/10.1186/s13148-021-01035-3
Aristotle. (1944). *Politics* (Vol. 1). (H. Rackham, Trans.). Harvard University Press. Retrieved June 2, 2022, from Perseus Catalogue: http://data.perseus.org/citations/urn:cts:greekLit:tlg0086.tlg035.perseus-eng1:1.1252b

Balibar, E. (1991). Is There a "Neo-Racism"? In E. Balibar & I. Wallerstein (Eds.), *Race, Nation, Class: Ambiguous Identities* (pp. 17–28). Verso.

Bederman, G. (1995). *Manliness and Civilization: A Cultural History of Gender and Race in the US 1880–1917.* Unversity of Chicago Press.

Bombay, A., Matheson, K., & Anisman, H. (2014). The Intergenerational Effects of Indian Residential Schools: Implications for the Concept of Historical Trauma. *Transcultural Psychiatry, 51*(3), 320–338.

Bourdieu, P. (1977). *Outline of a Theory of Practice.* (R. Nice, Trans.). Cambridge University Press.

Braun, L. (2002). Race, Ethnicity and Health – Can Genetics Explain Disparities. *Perspectives in Biology and Medicine, 45*(2), 159–174.

Braun, L. (2006). Reifying Human Difference: The Debate on Genetics, Race, and Health. *International Journal of Health Services, 36*(3), 55–73.

Brooks, B. (2022, October 2022). Philadelphia apologizes for experiments on Black inmates at Holmsburg Prison. Retrieved from 6abc Philadelphia: https://6abc.com/holmesburg-prison-experiments-philadelphia-apology-dr-albert-klingman-university-of-pennsylvania/12300722/

Clennon, O. D. (2016). The Black Face of Eurocentrism: Uncovering Globalisation. In O. D. Clennon (Ed.), *International Perspectives of Multiculturalism: The Ethical Challenges* (pp. 91–128). Nova Science Publishers.

Clennon, O. D. (2018). *Black Scholarly Activism Between the Academy and Grassroots: A Bridge for Identities and Social Justice.* Palgrave Macmillan.

Clennon, O. D. (2019, February 22). *Research in Social Justice: Why "Whiteness" Matters in the Real Word.* Retrieved June 1, 2022, from Palgrave Macmillan: https://www.palgrave.com/gp/campaigns/social-justice/ornette-clennon

Clennon, O. D. (2022, June 20). *Palgrave Studies in Decolonisation and Grassroots Black Organic Intellectualism (MaSPP).* Retrieved from MaCTRI (MEaP Academy Community Training and Research Institute): https://critracemmu.wordpress.com/decoloniality-in-the-grassroots-the-key-to-social-justice/

Cole, M. (2018, July 20). *The 'Strong Black Woman' Stereotype Is Harming Our Mental Health.* Retrieved from The Guardian. https://www.theguardian.com/commentisfree/2018/jul/20/strong-black-woman-stereotype-mental-health-depression-self-harm

Collins, P. H. (1990). *Black Feminist Thought.* Harper Collins.

Crenshaw, K. (1991). Mapping the Margins: Intersectionality, Identity Politics and Violence Against Women of Color. *Stanford Law Review, 43*(6), 1241–1299.

Curry, T. J. (2017). *THE MAN-NOT: Race, Class, Genre and the Dilemmas of Black Manhood.* Temple University Press.

Curry, T. J. (2021). Decolonising the Intersection. In R. K. Beshara (Ed.), *Critical Psychology Practice: Psychosocial Non-alignment to Modernity/Coloniality* (pp. 132–154). Routledge.

Curtis, L. A. (1975). *Violence, Race and Culture.* Lexington Book.

Curtis, L. A. (1976). Rape, Race and Culture: Some Speculations in Search of a Theory. In M. J. Walker & S. L. Brodsky (Eds.), *Sexual Assault: The Victim and the Rapist* (pp. 117–134). Lexington Books.

DeGruy Leary, J. (2005). *Post traumatic Slave Syndrome: America's Legacy of Enduring Injury and Healing.* Uptone Press.

Dunn, R. (1866). *Civilisation and Cerebral Development : Some Observations on the Influence of Civilisation Upon the Development of the Brain in the Different Races of Man.* Wellcome Collection. Available at https://wellcomecollection.org/works/qypmpny6

Equiano, O. (2005 [1789]). *The Interesting Narrative of the Life of Olaudah Equiano, or Gustavus Vassa, the African, Written by Himself.* (S. Shell, & D. Monico, Eds.). Project Gutenberg.

Evans-Campbell, T. (2008). Historical Trauma in American Indian/Native Alaska Communities: A Multilevel Framework for Exploring Impacts on Individuals, Families and Communities. *Journal of Interpersonal Violence, 23*(3), 316–338.

Fanon, F. (1986 [1952]). *Black Skin, White Masks.* (C. L. Markmann, Trans.). Pluto Press.

Fenton, K., Pawson, E., & Souza-Thomas, L. (2020). *Beyond the Data: Understanding the Impact of COVID-19 on BAME Communities.* Public Health England. Available at https://assets.publishing.service.gov.uk/government/uploads/system/uploads/attachment_data/file/892376/COVID_stakeholder_engagement_synthesis_beyond_the_data.pdf

Gamble, J., & McCallum, R. (2022). *Local Child Safeguarding Practice Review March 2022.* CHSCP. Available at https://chscp.org.uk/wp-content/uploads/2022/03/Child-Q-PUBLISHED-14-March-22.pdf

Garza, A. (2020, June 5). *Black Lives Matter: An Evening with Co-founder Alicia Garza.* Retrieved from CSUSM Library: https://csusm-dspace.calstate.edu/handle/10211.3/216449.

Geiger, H. J. (1981, June 21). An Experiment with Lives. Retrieved from *The New York Times*: https://archive.nytimes.com/www.nytimes.com/books/98/12/06/specials/jones-blood.html.

Graff, G. (2014). The Intergenerational Trauma of Slavery and Its Aftermath. *The Journal of Psychohistory, 41*(3), 181–197.

Griffin, S. (1971). An all-American Crime. *Ramparts, 10*(3), 26–56.

Grosfoguel, R. (2013). The Structure of Knowledge in Westernized Universities: Epistemic Racism/Sexism and the Four Genocides/Epistemicides of the Long 16th Century. *Human Architecture, 11*(1), 73–90.

Gyekye, K. (1995). *An Essay on African Philosophical Thought: The Akan Conceptual Scheme.* Temple University Press.

Hegel, G. (1977). *The Phenomenology of Spirit.* (A. V. Miller, Trans.). Clarendon Press.

Hegel, G. W. (1991). *The Philosophy of History.* (J. Sibree, Trans.). Prometheus Books.

Higginbotham, E. B. (1993). *Righteous Discontent: The Women's Movement in the Black Baptist Church, 1880–1920.* Harvard University Press.

Hoffman, K. M., Trawalter, S., Axt, J. R., & Oliver, M. N. (2016). Racial Bias in Pain Assessment and Treatment Recommendations and False Beliefs About Biological Differences Between Blacks and Whites. *Proceedings of the National Academy of Sciences of the United States of America, 113*(16), 4296–4301.

Hooks, B. (2004). *We Real Cool: Black Men and Masculinity.* Routledge.

Hooks, B., & West, C. (1999). *Breaking Bread: Insurgent Black Intellectual Life.* South End Press.

Hunt, J. (1863). *The Negro's Place in Nature.* Trubner. Available at https://openlibrary.org/books/OL33077648M/On_the_Negro%27s_place_in_nature

Jones, J. H. (1981 [1993]). *Bad Blood: The Tuskegee Syphillis Experiment.* The Free Press.

Jones, D. M. (2005). *Race, Sex and Suspicion: The Myth of the Black Male.* Praeger.

Kim, Y., Huan, T., Joehanes, R., McKeown, N. M., Horvath, S., Levy, D., & Ma, J. (2022). Higher Diet Quality Relates to Decelerated Epigenetic Aging. *The American Journal of Clinical Nutrition, 115*(1), 163–170.

Knight, M. (2019). The Findings of the MBRRACE-UK Confidential Enquiry into Maternal Deaths and Morbidity. *Obstetrics, Gynaecology and Reproductive Medicine, 29*(1), 21–23.

Laqueur, T. W. (1990). *Making Sex. Body and Gender from the Greeks to Freud.* Harvard University Press.

Long, J. (2022, August 8). Exclusive: Medics treated arrested man 'like he was pretending' before seizure death, says family. Retrieved from Channel4 News: https://www.channel4.com/news/exclusive-medics-treated-arrested-man-like-he-was-pretending-before-seizure-death-says-family

Lugones, M. (2008). The Coloniality of Gender. *Worlds and Knowledges Otherwise, 2*(Spring), 1–17.

MacKinnon, C. A. (1989). *Toward a Feminist Theory of the State*. Harvard University Press.

Maldonado-Torres, N. (2007). On the Coloniality of Being: Contributions to the Development of a Concept. *Cultural Studies (London, England), 21*(2–3), 240–270.

Mbiti, J. S. (1970). *African Religions and Philosophy*. Anchor Books.

McGinley, K. F., Tay, K. J., & Moul, J. W. (2016). Prostate Cancer in Men of African Origin. *Nature Reviews Urology, 13*(2), 99–107.

Michelet, J. (1867). *Woman (La Femme)*. (J. W. Palmer, Trans.). Carleton.

Mignolo, W. (2000). *Local Histories/Global Designs: Essays on the Coloniality of Power, Subaltern Knowledges and Border Thinking*. Princeton University Press.

Mignolo, W. (2002). The Geopolitics of Knowledge and the Colonial Difference. *South Atlantic Quarterly, 101*(1), 57–96.

Mignolo, W. D., & Escobar, A. (Eds.). (2010). *Globalization and the Decolonial Option*. Routledge.

Newman, L. M. (1999). *WHITE WOMEN'S RIGHTS: The Racial Origins of Feminism in the United States*. Oxford University Press.

Odedina, F. T., Yu, D., Akinremi, T. O., Reams, R. R., Freedman, M. L., & Kumar, N. (2009). Prostate Cancer Cognitive-Behavioural Factors in a West African Population. *Journal of Immigrant and Minority Health, 11*(4), 258–267.

Ogbu, J. (2004). Collective Identity and the Burden of "Acting White" in Black History, Community, and Education. *The Urban Review, 36*(1), 1–35.

Oruka, H. O. (1990). *Sage Philosophy: Indigenous Thinkers and Modern Debate on African Philosophy*. E. J. Brill.

Oyěwùmí, O. (1997). *The Invention of Women: Making an African Sense of Western Gender Discourses*. University of Minneapolis Press.

Paul, R. (2009). "I Whitened My Face, That They Might Not Know Me": Race and Identity in Olaudah Equiano's Slave Narrative. *Journal of Black Studies, 36*(9), 848–864.

Payne-Sturges, D. C., Gee, G. C., & Cory-Slechta, D. A. (2021). Confronting Racism in Environmental Health Sciences: Moving the Science Forward for Eliminating Racial Inequities. *Environmental Health Perspectives, 129*(5). https://doi.org/10.1289/EHP8186

Prather, C., Fuller, T. R., Jeffries, W. L., IV, Marshall, K. J., Howell, A. V., Belyue-Umole, A., & King, W. (2018). *Health Equity, 2*(1), 249–259. Available at https://www.liebertpub.com/doi/10.1089/heq.2017.0045

Quijano, A. (2007). Coloniality And Modernity/Rationality. *Cultural Studies, 21*(2–3), 168–178.

Rebbeck, T. R., Devesa, S. S., Chang, B.-L., Bunker, C. H., Cheng, I., Cooney, K., et al. (2013, February 13). *Global Patterns of Prostate Cancer Incidence, Aggressiveness, and Mortality in Men of African Descent.*

Robinson, C. (1983). *Black Marxism: The Making of the Black Radical Tradition.* Zed Press.

Rose, W. L. (1982). In W. W. Freehlint (Ed.), *Slavery and Freedom.* Oxford University Press.

Rosenthal, L., & Lobel, M. (2016). Stereotypes of Black American Women Related to Sexuality and Motherhood. *Psychology of Women Quarterly, 40*(3), 414–427.

Sefa Dei, G. (2014). Indigenizing the Curriculum: The Case of the African University. In G. Emeagwali & G. Sefa Dei (Eds.), *African Indigenous Knowledge and the Disciplines* (pp. 165–180). Sense Publishers.

Shackel, P. A. (2018). Transgenerational Impact of Structural Violence: Epigenetics and the Legacy of Anthracite Coal. *International Journal of Historical Archaeology, 22*(4), 865–882.

The Met. (2022, March 25). *Strip search data.* Retrieved from Mayor of London: London Assembly: https://www.london.gov.uk/questions/2022/0501.

Tosh, J. (2016). *Manliness and Masculinities in Nineteenth–Century Britain: Essays on Gender, Family and Empire.* Routledge. Retrieved June 12, 2022, from https://www.perlego.com/book/1552790/manliness-and-masculinities-in-nineteenthcentury-britain-pdf

Walter, D. (2016). *Colonial Violence: European Empires and the Use of Force.* (P. Lewis, Trans.). Oxford University Press.

Wells-Barnett, I. B. (2014 [1892]). *On Lynchings.* Dover Publications.

Williams, D. R., Lawrence, J. A., Davis, B. A., & Vu, C. (2019). Understanding How Discrimination Can Affect Health. *Health Services Research, 54*(S2), 1374–1388.

Wollstonecraft, M. (2002 [1792]). *A Vindication of the Rights of Woman Title: Vindication of the Rights of Women.* (S. Tomaselli, Ed.). Project Gutenberg Literary Archive Foundation.

4

Decolonising Public Health: What Are the Alternatives?

Abstract In this chapter, we will look at "traditional health knowledges" in UK African Diaspora grassroots communities. We will also discuss whether a Eurocentric view of health is compatible with a more Afrocentric framework of holistic health (i.e. the integration between mind, body and spirit). Using Ubuntu's (see an African Philosophy to Education c.f. Waghid & Smeyers, Educational Philosophy and Theory, 44(S2), 6–20, 2012) ethno-philosophical framework (Emeagwali, Intersections Between Africa's Indigenous Knowledge Systems and History. In G. Emeagwali, & G. Sefa Dei (Eds.), African Indigenous Knowledge and the Disciplines (pp. 1–19). Sense Publishers, 2014; Sefa Dei, Indigenizing the Curriculum: The Case of the African University. In G. Emeagwali, & G. Sefa Dei (Eds.), African Indigenous Knowledge and the Disciplines (pp. 165–180). Sense Publishers, 2014) and critical philosophy (Gyekye, An Essay on African Philosophical Thought: The Akan Conceptual Scheme. Temple University Press, 1995; Dzobo, African Symbols and Proverbs as Sources of Knowledge. In K. Wiredu, & K. Gyekye (Eds.), Person and Community: Ghanaian Philosophical Studies I (Vol. 1) (pp. 85–98). Council for Research in Values and Philosophy, 1992) as

---

The original version of the chapter has been revised. A correction to this chapter can be found at https://doi.org/10.1007/978-3-031-18405-5_6

79

F. Bruce, O. D. Clennon, *Decolonising Public Health through Praxis*, https://doi.org/10.1007/978-3-031-18405-5_4

starting points, we will attempt to excavate traditional epistemologies around health that revolve around pre-colonial ontologies of community. To do this, we will listen to the voices of our community members to glean nuggets of intergenerational cultural wisdoms about alternative models of health, as we examine the influence of the Black Church (both Caribbean-led and African-led) on health. Finally, we will look at how Church leaders can play a larger role in mediating access to the health market for their congregations in order to achieve better health outcomes.

Keywords Holistic health • Traditional health epistemologies • Black Church • African metaphysics

Introduction

The Importance of the Church for Health Support

Faye: My dad was a Deacon in a large church that he was privileged to help establish not long after they arrived from Jamaica. Most of the congregants in the church were from Jamaica and came to our house sharing fond memories of being back home in Jamaica. In fact, the church was the sanctuary, and it was the place people went for not only spiritual fulfilment but also for social, economic and physical support.

Ornette: Yes, the Church has indeed played a significant role in supporting newly arrived migrants from the Caribbean as I can also see that in my family, for whom church still remains important.

F: I remember when I was around ten years old, I overheard one of mum and dad's friends weeping in the kitchen having recently lost his wife. Finding it difficult to contain his emotions he spoke about the difficulty his wife had when she went to get help from the GP. He said that time and time again she would visit the GP saying that she wasn't feeling well but yet they did nothing but repeatedly send her away without checking or referring her for another opinion. Mum and dad's friend died in her sleep only two days after visiting the GP. She was only forty years old and left behind six young children. Several stories of this nature where people had died, had amputations in their forties due to unmanaged diabetes were overheard. It was so traumatic for me as a young child along with my siblings sometimes going with mum and dad to visit people in hospital and subsequently attend their funerals. I remember being taken along with my siblings to all night wakes in the home or relative you visited of the person that had died. Friends and family members would sing hymns until the early hours of the morning supporting the family. Some of mum and dad's friends died young (early to mid-forties) and I was so anxious about my own parents and what would happen to them.

O: This sounds very much like a continuation of the institutional neglect you described earlier.[1]

F: Definitely! The stressors were phenomenal for my parents who have paid the price with their own health. They were fortunate to have a good network of friends from church and in Jamaica. They were devoted Christians who would spend a lot of time in prayer and bible reading, which they said gave them comfort and strength at night especially after we had heard of a passing. At those times, I could not sleep and decades later I am still mindful of these formative events. It is only now in my later years that I begin to see the impact that the personal and social stressors that this 'work harder' ethic had on both my mum and many of her friends as they fought against racial, economic and gender oppressions that confined them to certain roles and positions in society.

Commentary

In our various conversations with members of our communities mainly from Jamaica, Barbados, a few smaller Caribbean Islands, Nigeria and Ghana they regularly tell us about the lack of value attached to their cultural needs and their religious practices and beliefs (MaCTRI, 2017b). They also speak about how their cultural practices are extremely important especially in relation to their health and coping strategies when treating illness. Billingsley (1999) argues that religion and the church act as buffers and play a key role in helping to build the resilience of Black people who are oppressed by the legacies of whiteness. Perdue et al. (2006) also found that spirituality often provides emotional consolation,

---

[1] See Chap. 3.

inspiration and guidance whilst fostering personal responsibility, identity and community building. Echoing this, Nguyen et al. (2019, pp. discussion, para 7) observed that "church members [can] act as surrogate family to individuals who lack family ties".

Mbiti (1970, p. 136) describes a pre-colonial (traditional) African echo of these church relationships as:

> The kinship system is like a vast network stretching laterally (horizontally) in every direction, to embrace everybody in any given local group. This means that each individual is a brother or sister, father or mother, grandmother or grandfather, or cousin, or brother in-law, uncle or aunt, or something else, to everybody else. That means that everybody is related to everybody else.

Many of our community partners are members of Black-led churches.[2] And many of the churches that our community partners attend are Pentecostal churches. According to Burrell (2019, p. 34):

> Pentecostals believe that faith must be powerfully experiential, and not something found merely through ritual or thinking. Pentecostalism is energetic and dynamic. Its members believe they are driven by the power of God moving within them. Pentecostal churches stress the importance of conversions through Baptism in the Spirit. This fills the believer with the Holy Spirit, which gives the believer the strength to live a truly Christian life. The direct experience of God is revealed by gifts of the Spirit, such as speaking in tongues, prophecy and healing. Pentecostal Christians accept the status of The Bible as the indisputable and irrefutable Word of God.

The description of Pentecostalism above gives us another tantalising echo of traditional African religions. Mbiti (1970, p. 4) tells us that

> The whole environment and the whole time must be occupied by religious meaning, so that at any moment and in any place, a person feels secure enough to act in a meaningful and religious consciousness.

---

[2] See Burrell (2019) for discussion about the nuanced differences between Black majority churches with 50 percent or more Black members in the UK but having white majority parent churches abroad and Black-led churches both nationally and internationally.

Mbiti (1970) explains that across the African Continent, religion denotes a way of life and being for tribal life. Each tribe has its own religious traditions that it uses to cohere and unify its kinship networks and these religious traditions are not transferable across tribes although similarities in belief systems might exist. The most important facet of African religions that Mbiti stresses is that it is all consuming in terms of bonding the individual to their community. Religion for such an individual is a constant and active process of "being" that is not necessarily contained by rituals or worship at appointed times in the week. We would say that this fundamental element of African religions is what could have perhaps attracted many of our African communities to Pentecostalism, as the latter also requires an active process of "being" in the Holy Spirit to live a Christian life.[3, 4]

One of our community partners alludes to this:

Faith and religion cannot be one without the other—you see me? Then you see my faith through my religious practices.

However, the kinship of Church and the Pentecostal bonding with the Holy Spirit in Black churches also very much reminds us of a pre-colonial

---

[3] Burrell (2019, p. 32) provides a good account of the rise of Pentecostalism in the UK that involved the Rev. Kwame Brem-Wilson (1906–1929) a Ghanaian businessman who "became the first African Pentecostal leader at Sumner Road Chapel in Peckham, South East London".

[4] However, it is also important to note that

Christianity in Africa is so old that it can rightly be described as an indigenous, traditional and African religion. Long before the start of Islam in the seventh century, Christianity was well established all over north Africa, Egypt, parts of the Sudan and Ethiopia. It was a dynamic form of Christianity, producing great scholars and theologians like Tertullian, Origen, Clement of Alexandria and Augustine. African Christianity made a great contribution to Christendom through scholarship, participation in Church councils, defence of the Faith, movements like monasticism, theology, translation and preservation of the Scriptures, martyrdom, the famous Catechetical School of Alexandria, liturgy and even heresies and controversies. (Mbiti, 1970, p. 300)

African sense of community, which today is encapsulated in Ubuntu's[5] apho-rism, "I am because we/you are". Mbiti (1970, p. 141) describes this as:

> What then is the individual and where is his place in the community? In traditional life, the individual does not and cannot exist alone except corporately. He owes his existence to other people, including those of past generations and his contemporaries. He is simply part of the whole. The community must therefore make, create or produce the individual; for the individual depends on the corporate group.

Harmon et al. (2018, p. 1513) echo this feeling of kinship in their study:

> The congregation looked to [pastors] for more. A pastor in an African-American church was far more than … someone who teaches and preaches. If you go back to African culture, you're almost a tribal leader, and so that tradition sort of continues.

As regards the immense influence of the pastor on their congregation, Heward-Mills et al. (2018, pp. discussion, para 5) observed in their study that:

> Faith leaders have been known to have immense authority within the church and to use this to promote positive health behaviour. Some participants in the study actually described faith leader as some sort of Demi God who is so revered and influential, that they cannot be wrong and are even worshipped by some congregants.

Cultural and religious beliefs impact upon health decisions and these decisions create barriers to the health market as the way in which the health system is set up denies the reality of Black people's traditional practices, for example, not engaging in IVF because of a conflict between

---

[5] Clennon (2018, p. 82)

Ubuntu is a South African Zulu term that denotes "human kindness" or "humaneness". Ubuntu seeks to examine the relationship between the individual and their community.

beliefs in God and the role of medicine. Also, sometimes there being the idea that some health conditions are related to witchcraft,[6] often leading to people feeling ostracised and isolated. In our conversations, we have found that the church is not always a place where people find refuge because of stigmatising conditions where people are deemed not to have enough faith if they rely on western diagnosis and medication. Our community partners refer to how some conditions such as mental illness and diseases such as cancer and HIV are thought to be brought about by curses, making the community uncomfortable discussing them. However, in their study, Nunn et al. (2012, pp. discussion, para 4) report that:

> [t]here was a common consensus that discussing controversial topics such as HIV/AIDS was easier for more established faith leaders with larger followings and more experience. This suggests that engaging more experienced pastors to help jumpstart public dialogue about HIV/AIDS might help normalize discussions about HIV/AIDS with the faith community.

The stigma often prevents engagement with health services to address the condition. This poses an interesting question about the extent to which the Black Church can become a site of decolonial agency (towards improved health outcomes for its members) considering its colonial origins. However, in terms of building resilience, faith leaders undoubtedly have been and continue to be influential in motivating others in church congregations to take more responsibility for their health (Heward-Mills et al. 2018; Gross et al. 2018).

Our community members tell us about their affiliations to culture and/or religion which provides them with a sense of "belonging, purpose and confidence" but also where within that group they can self-identify and define who they are. They often speak about the trust they have towards each other because they have the same values and beliefs, which is especially pertinent from a religious perspective.

In our conversations, the faith of many of our community partners is so strong that they rely only on their faith to be healed. One community member tells us that they were told by their General Practitioner (GP) that they had depression and anxiety and that they needed to take

---

[6] See note 11.

medication to help them. Even though they took the prescription they never had the medicine dispensed, they said:

> depression, depression, what depression, that is not of God, I rebuke it!

Casarez and Miles (2008) note that the women in their study believed that God was in control and that God required an active relationship with Him, which resulted in apparent reductions in anxiety of about their health and that of their children.[7] However, for some of our community members, this prevents them from engaging effectively with health services. In Caribbean and African communities, our partners tell us that it is often the case that when people become unwell, they engage the services of a traditional healer or faith leader for healing that often involves the use of herbal remedies.

A community partner tells us:

> Every day when I wake up in the morning I pray and have faith that God will take me through the often-stressful challenges of the day, when I say stressful these may be financial. When I was back in Africa 30 years ago, we did not have doctors like here [UK] we had traditional healers, they were sent as doctors and we believed that God would use these people to protect us from getting mentally ill.

Commentary

African Healers[8]

Some of our community partners tell us that they often visited local traditional healers for assistance with their health needs, when they were back home in Africa.

---

[7] We must remember that prayer is a well-known (if little understood) healing phenomenon, globally (e.g. Johnson, 2018; Newitt, 2022; Akbari et al., 2020; Friedrich-Killinger, 2020; Miranda et al., 2020; Romez et al., 2021; Abu et al., 2019; Brown, 2012; Maier-Lorentz, 2004; Levin, 2009, etc.).

[8] Also see Clennon (2022a) for similar collaborative work in a Brazilian shamanic context with the Tukano people from the Amazonian rainforest.

Who Are the Traditional Healers?

Mbiti (1970, pp. 217–218) explains that:

To African societies the medicine-men are the greatest gift, and the most useful source of help. Other names for them are "herbalists," "traditional doctors" or "waganga" (to use a Swahili word). These are the specialists who have suffered most from European-American writers and speakers who so often and wrongly call them "witch-doctors"—a term which should be buried and forgotten forever. Every village in Africa has a medicine-man within reach, and he is the friend of the community. He is accessible to everybody and at almost all times, and comes into the picture at many points in individual and community life.

What Do Traditional Healers Do?

Medicine-men and women undergo formal and informal training according to their tribal customs. Their training that can last many years, if they are trained from childhood, incorporates knowledge of the medicinal properties found in their local flora. They also need to be trained in divination. Divination, as we will discuss later, is crucial for the African healer to be able to discern the spiritual causes of illness.

Sogolo (2003, p. 235) tells us that:

Unlike the modern physician who has to rely almost entirely on the pharmacological efficacy of drugs, cure for the traditional African healer is directed towards the two targets of primary and secondary causes. The healer may be confident of the pharmacological activities of his/her herbs, but that is not all. The herbs are efficacious, the healer believes, only if the primary causes have been taken care of. The herbalist is thus also a diviner, which gives his/her profession a metaphysical outlook. But, again, this could be misleading. The point is that the primary causes result in the weakening of the defence mechanisms of the body. Cure in this respect simply means restoring the body to a state of increased capacity to heal itself, a state in which the pharmacological efficacy of the drugs is maximized.

Mbiti (1970, p. 221) expands on this:

This is the process that medicine-men follow in dealing with illness and misfortune: it is partly psychological and partly physical. Thus, the medicine-man applies both physical and "spiritual" (or psychological) treatment, which assures the sufferer that all is and will be well. The medicine-man is in effect both doctor and pastor to the sick person.

Both Sogolo (2003) and Mbiti (1970) write about the "metaphysical" and "spiritual" in describing healing. We think that it is important to briefly outline the philosophical context within which these frameworks reside in order to better understand the function of the African healer.

African Religions

We touched on the centrality of religion to pre-colonial (traditional) communities and its contemporary echoes with Pentecostalism. So, let's briefly explore the basic principles of African religions, as this will give context to the role and function of the African healer. Mbiti (1970, p. 38) tells us that:

In all these societies, without a single exception, people have a notion of God as the Supreme Being. This is the most minimal and fundamental idea about God, found in all African societies.

This is important to remember about African spirituality, as it is a point that has been often lost on colonial outsiders.[9] Asante and Mazama (2009, pp. 20th century re-discovery of African Religions, para. 9) expand on this:

What is believed intensely all over the continent of Africa is that the Supreme Being, who could be male, female, or both, created the universe, animals, and human beings, but soon retreated from any direct involve-

---

[9] See Chap. 3 and Hegel for his Sepúlveda complex concerning his perceived Godlessness of the "Negro", especially ironic for his seeming ignorance of Africa's shaping of the very Christian religion that he esteemed as being superior. See note 4.

ment in the affairs of humans. In some cases in Africa, the Supreme Being does not finish the creation; it is left to other deities to complete. Among the Yoruba, this delegation of creation appears when Olorun, the Owner of the Sky, the Supreme God, starts the creation of the universe and then leaves it to Obatala, a lesser deity, to complete the task. Among the Herero of Namibia, the Supreme God, Omukuru, the Great One, Njambi Kurunga, withdrew into the sky after creating lesser divinities and humans. There are neither temples nor shrines to the God of Gods among most people in Africa. In most cases, the lesser divinities are worshipped, revered, loved, and feared.

The above quote is important because the metaphysical or spiritual aspect of indigenous African faith is centred around the unseen interactions between the Supreme Being, the lesser divinities sent to finish their work of creation, (the spirits of) ancestors and human beings. In African spirituality, everyone is acculturated to see the physical world simultaneously with the spiritual world where its "unseen" processes produce effects in the physical world. Because the Supreme Being in many tribal customs is a remote figure, their emissaries or intermediaries gain importance in bridging the gap between the spiritual and physical worlds, as managed by the healers (specialists).

However, to make sense of what constitutes the spiritual world, we will briefly need to outline the African concept of time. Mbiti (1970) explains that the pre-colonial (traditional) African sense of time is roughly divided into two categories; Sasa and Zamani (Swahili words that Mbiti chooses as being representative across Black Africa to illustrate the African concept of time). Sasa refers to the present—but an extended present that incorporates the very recent past and the immediate future. Mbiti calls this "Micro Time" (p. 28). In essence, the traditional African mind only recognises events that have been recently experienced, being experienced (now) or about to be experienced (up to two years in advance) personally by the speaker. Mbiti explains that within Sasa, time is measured by events or landmark happenings not by actual chronology. It is expected that these events will roughly fall within a specific chronological marker (such as Spring) but it is the event itself that is important not its chronology. So, Sasa is about a *personal* experience of time. Also, important to note that further than two years in the future does not really exist in African chronology as it falls too far outside personal experience.[10] So, because there is no distant future, it is the past or the distant past that becomes supremely important and this is called Zamani or "Macro Time" (p. 29). Mbiti explains that Zamani is a distant past that the speaker has no personal access to (so, beyond their Sasa), a past where memories and myths reside, a past that acts as a repository for all that has passed. Both Sasa and Zamani are interlinked, where Zamani provides stability for Sasa and both have their own conceptual forms in terms of size and even tense! For us, this means that both Sasa and Zamani form "actual" (living) places on metaphysical or spiritual planes in the African

---

[10] This is interesting to us because it means that within this African metaphysical framework, progress as a continual striving for and into the future is alien to the average traditional African thinker. For them, what is important is honouring their past and how that past makes them who they are in the "now". For us, this is a profound distinguishing feature of African metaphysics that sits in opposition to Eurocentric philosophical traditions that form the basis of the Western preoccupation with growth and progress (futurity). It would appear that without a sufficiently deep and textured knowledge of one's history, it becomes difficult to appreciate what one has and this lack of grounding can lead to the intense desire of wanting more (mastery). This can happen at both personal and national levels (where synthetic and pragmatic narratives of national unity, do not count as "deep and textured knowledge" of one's history see Clennon (2016b)). Also see Clennon (2016a) for a psychoanalytical take on this drive of whiteness that is based on futurity. African metaphysics seems to avoid all of this with its focus on a Sasa that is grounded by Zamani.

On the other hand, the apparent lack of historical introspection that characterises Western/Eurocentric metaphysics is closely related to the Sepúlveda complex where this profound lack of reflexive capacity prevents the Western observer from really seeing the "now" that they are presented with because they are blinded by their prejudices (that consist of specious ideologies revolving around "progress" or civility, as well as their own disavowed immoralities) driven by *their* metaphysical plane of futurity, which also has emissaries who straddle the now and the future. Emissaries? For examples, think of neoliberal markets in general (including the exchange-traded derivative contracts comprising the Futures market) and venture capitalists in particular investing in start-ups whose value lies in their future not their present. Also see Clennon (2016a) for analysis of how whiteness acts as a market derivative. These capitalist ideas around future-projection might not be personified like entities residing in Sasa and Zamani but they are no less impactful on the Western mind from their residence in futurity! (i.e. capitalist (futurist) ideologies are near-deified in terms of our current world order, as brilliantly personified in Neil Gaiman's *American Gods*! (Gaiman, 2004). In fact, specialists (also known as bankers in this context) of manipulating emissaries from this metaphysical plane of futurity have even been dubbed the new "Masters of the Universe" (Diessner & Lisi, 2020, p. 315), a development of McGee's (2010, p. 129) verbatim reference to transnational corporations. See note 11 for a direct comparison with African specialists). We would go as far as to suggest that this obsession with futurity is what lies behind the West's preoccupation with erasing/rewriting the past in favour of a constantly reinvented and self serving/centring present (Nora, 1996) (for profit) that is always inflected by futurity. Of course, we already recognise whiteness' preoccupation with erasing the past in its guise of the many epistemicides and genocides it has waged over the centuries (De Sousa Santos, 2010; Dussel, 2000)!

mind, that are populated by various entities (e.g. recently passed ancestors). This means that everything (e.g. knowledge and traditions) is kept alive "in spirit" by passing from Sasa into Zamani. Death in this African context is when those memories no longer exist in Zamani.

So, in African metaphysics, when someone dies, they live on in the Sasa of their relatives and communities and Mbiti describes this as a "personal immortality" (Mbiti, 1970, p. 32), where they are remembered by name. This means that they are not really dead but alive in the minds of those who survived them; they are known as "living dead" (p. 32). Sasa remembrance is also kept alive through relatives and their children and children's children, and so on. So, offering a libation or food to a dead ancestor is an act of remembrance rather than worship. When the "living dead" fall out of the Sasa into Zamani, where there are no longer any living memories of them (i.e. their direct survivors have all died), they then achieve "collective immortality" (p. 33) where they are remembered collectively by a community but not in a personal Sasa way but more in a mythological Zamani manner. Mbiti says at this point, that their name becomes "empty" (p. 34), as there is no longer a personal connection. However, the deceased finally achieves real death when they are no longer remembered in Zamani. So alongside lesser deities, ancestors who reside in both Sasa and Zamani are thought to be able to act as emissaries between the spiritual and physical worlds.

It is beyond the scope of this chapter to give details on the various roles and functions of such emissaries, as this is extremely well documented by Asante & Mazama's (2009) *Encyclopedia of African Religion* and also Sutherland's et al. (2014) *Caribbean Healing Traditions* for the healing and religious system of Obeah in the Caribbean. But it is important to note that occurrences in the physical world such as health will be viewed as also having a spiritual origin[11] that will also need to be acknowledged. So, within this physical and spiritual metaphysical framework, where coincidence and chance cannot exist (in Sasa or Zamani), the African healer (specialist) needs to be adept at navigating between these two worlds in order to diagnose and treat the causes of illness.

---

[11] Such as, for example, an ancestor taking offence at not being honoured or someone (usually a specialist from the physical world) manipulating emissaries to do harm to someone else in the physical world; sometimes known as witchcraft. In this case a diviner/healer (specialist) would use charms and potions to protect their client/patient from the effects of the spiritual attack.

Health Prevention (i.e. Disease Prevention)

The gap in health prevention information often leads us to discuss issues around trust and how it features when engaging the community, especially when information does not address them or consider their overall cultural needs in health prevention and guidance.

One community member tells us:

> It has been really difficult recently because we lost another sister in the church and you know, there is a part of me that blames the health service for many of the people we have lost; people dying from things like diabetes when it may have just needed some health information directed at us.

One of our community members held some very strong perceptions about the lack of trust from mainstream service providers[12] admits:

> I am not one that will go to the health service to get my information because the way Black people are treated doesn't allow me to trust them, I turn to my church leader and I can then make sense of whatever they tell me or direct me too.

Another community partner tells us:

> Back home in Jamaica, everything that was there was about you, they [health professionals] got it, they were familiar, and it was well intended. There were no differences in treatment [may be a little issue with manners] even then, they understood how to treat you.

Gross, et al. (2018, pp. discussion, para 6) notes that in their study, in order to try to address this issue of mistrust the:

> Pastors were hopeful that younger women would begin new traditions of health and fitness, passing it along to their families. As leaders in the Black church, women have the ability to greatly influence health for themselves, families, and communities.

---

[12] See Chaps. 2 and 3 for details about some of those reasons for mistrust.

In Caribbean and African communities, faith and culture are often the common denominator in decision-making about health due to their pastors often having a holistic approach to health that integrated spirituality in their perspectives (Williams & Cousin, 2021). Sogolo (2003, p. 233) reminds us of the origins of this approach in our communities:

> The firm assumption has always been that African cultures hold a holistic conception of disease or illness people are considered ill if they display a state of unusual feeling, suffering pain or incapacitation, or being in danger of death or mutilation. Once day-to-day life activities (e.g. the ability to work or to perform other social duties) are affected by this general feeling, such a person is said to be ill, whether or not the causes are traceable to specific structural changes in the cells of the body.

However, some of our partners tell us that they believed that God provided doctors and other health professionals to be the tool used to help them in their treatment:

> My faith is so important to me, I would always commence with prayer before going to use hospital services when ill, sometimes I have a word from God that orders me to stay home and pray instead of going to use health services.

Traditional Remedies

African diasporic traditional medicines have been used as a form of protection from sickness and disease for decades. It is also used as a way of healing as there is often the belief that disease does not happen by chance but from ritual practices. In essence, this belief system is in conflict with western medical practice because the latter is more accepting of sickness and disease. This is illustrated by the idea that a General Practitioner (GP) can diagnose a condition that due to the patient's faith, is not recognised by them because they see it as originating from a spiritual source, which in turn is not recognised by the GP.

However, there is a wealth of literature (e.g. van Andel et al., 2012; Erwin & Peters, 1999; Carney, 2003; Mackenzie et al., 2003; George, 2012; Higginbottom & Mathers, 2006; Omodara et al., 2021, etc.) to highlight how people from the Caribbean and African community turn to traditional remedies in place of western medicine. It is often the case that Black people will adopt this option prior to engaging with their primary care provider when they have signs and symptoms of ill health. Even though many people (especially older people in our communities) come from Africa and the Caribbean islands where they had the opportunity to access western medicine, they were still keen to explore the traditional route to treat their illness. Scott (2010) also reminds us that primary care using western medicine can often be too expensive to access for health seekers in developing countries, hence the need for traditional alternatives. Our community partners often tell us about how doctors are hasty to treat a common complaint with medication when they believe that there are other options that they are familiar within their home countries. A community member tells us:

Medication is my last resort.
A community elder agrees
… and mi too, mi not taking dem for me to feel worse dan me feel already.

Some in our communities often speak about the unwanted treatments and recommendations for health problems that they see as being too harsh for their complaints. They often tell us, "we aren't talking pills: it's all about the natural remedies here".
When talking about his children, a partner says:

when they got a little cold or something like that, I would rub them up with the bay rum[13] and give them something to drink from the bush and that would be the end of it. All of them is good.

Faye: Our partners' accounts take me back to my childhood days when either my siblings or I were unwell. In fact, the thing that made you fearful and apprehensive was the thought of having to drink the bitter boiled bush tea that mum and dad gave to us. Our community partner is right … that bay rum, I can smell it now and how much better you would actually feel, amazing stuff!

---

[13] Used as a rubbing alcohol to relieve muscle soreness.

Commentary

Overall, our community members complain about how their cultural roots and assets are ignored despite the direct impact upon their health outcomes in terms of the level of poor, culturally insensitive healthcare provision and the inadequate health prevention guidance that they receive.

The African Model of Health

Asante and Mazama (2009, pp. Health, para. 1):

> Health in the African context refers to a state of positive mental and physical well-being. It is a state of normalcy marked by the absence of disease. The World Health Organization holds that health is a state of complete physical, mental, and social well-being and not merely the absence of disease or infirmity. Health may also be considered as a positive state necessary for the maintenance of physical and spiritual well-being. From this perspective, Africans see health as the normal state in which individuals can attain their best, thereby contributing toward the greater social good. Health is also understood as a state of well-being. Well-being refers to the state of fulfilment whereby both the individual and society are spared from mental and physical discomfort and enjoy peace of mind.

The above quote is significant for its foregrounding the importance of *well-being*. However, because African Diaspora health seekers traditionally "see health as a normal state", the crucial question that they ask of their ill health is "why am I ill?" (Scott, 2010, p. 86). Not what their illness is. The answers for this, as we have already discussed, lie deeply entwined in cultural beliefs, where the concept of well-being needs to be broken down into physical, mental, spiritual and social components, *if* their view of health is to be understood. If statutory providers are unable to recognise the holistic needs of these communities and are equally unable to work in real partnerships with them to achieve better understandings of their health epistemologies, this will inevitably foster mistrust.

Mistrust

In our conversations, our community partners often talk about the way in which Black people have often found themselves to suffer worse discrimination in everything and that as a consequence, they don't trust the intentions of health system. Community partners often complain about how society or what they describe as "the big wide world" does not respect or understand them or their culture, so gathering together with like-minded people is an important and reassuring protective factor for them. A partner tells us:

> This is about people understanding who you are, what you represent, this is important for our own sanity, our own views on illness and health are influenced by our culture and what our parents have brought us up to believe. When mum said to gwan chop up and boil the Chaney root[14] and drink it, that is exactly what you did … family and community [some community] is so important a central agent in caring for our mental wellbeing.

Our community members often talk about their mistrust in health professionals and although this is not about the health professionals themselves, they are more concerned about the way in which Black people are diagnosed by the system. They are also concerned about the way in which treatments are allocated to them without a full understanding about them and their cultural and religious response to illness.

Another community member expresses their mistrust of western medicine:

> What can we do in terms of coupling supplements for our bodies to be able to acclimatise in all areas like the lack of sun with vitamin D deficiency as we are not meant to be in such cold climates, this is curtailed and tested on people. Pharmaceuticals do not test on *our* people. We are not included and [are] benchmarked against [the] white majority.[15]

---

[14] Chaney Root is a traditional Jamaican herbal remedy for amongst other things; cleansing the blood, helping with arthritis and combatting fatigue. It is usually boiled and drunk as a tea.
[15] See Chap. 2 about benchmarking.

Another partner tells us:

What is the point of taking them; they have no idea how it is going to work on me because they haven't tested it on people that look like me. All I hear about are the side effects that people get, the fact is, you go to the doctor with one thing and come out with something else.[16]

Community members are keen to understand the real benefits and properties of their traditional remedies and many talk about how these remedies have cured many ills in the past. One of our community elders suggests that:

Research is needed into own cultural herbal remedies rather than just offered western medicines.

Another one of our older community members explains:

There is no such thing better that the stuff we get back home, none of this rubbish synthetic stuff you have here can treat us Black people. You see, whenever we have pain, belly ache and all of dat we just get addy Bissy or Cerasee[17] and just boil it up and drink it. We never did need fi visit addi doctor, our natural environment was our medicine.

Commentary

What lessons from the African Model of Health can we apply to 21st Century Grassroots Community Health Practices in the UK?

Before looking at the lessons that can be applied to grassroots health (disease) prevention, we will first need to briefly look at the international landscape for the use of traditional medicines. The World Health

---

[16] See Chap. 5 about genomic testing for better pharmaceutical drug-efficacy.

[17] A traditional medicinal herbal remedy native to Africa and used by Black people to improve overall general health and help to purge or cleanse the blood. Can be spelt as cerrasee or serasee. It is usually boiled and drunk as a tea. Bissy is a traditional medicinal herb remedy native to Jamaica (originally brought over from Nigeria) and is used by Black people for various ailments including relieving constipation, respiratory issues and mental well-being. It is usually boiled and drunk as a tea.

Organisation (WHO) at the United Nations has recognised the need for and has been working on a global strategy for better support and investment in traditional complementary medicines (T&CM), since 2002. The WHO recognises that T&CMs have and continue to be used worldwide either as primary care in rural communities in developing countries or as complementary medicine in developed countries with robust primary care systems. The following excerpts are taken from the WHO (2013) report that outlines its global priorities for T&CM and the WHO (2019) progress report where the state of play regarding T&CM in the United Kingdom is reported.

International Context: Traditional Medicine, WHO

WHO (2013, pp. 10–11):

> Traditional medicine (TM) is an important and often underestimated part of health services. In some countries, traditional medicine or non-conventional medicine may be termed complementary medicine (CM). TM has a long history of use in health maintenance and in disease prevention and treatment, particularly for chronic disease.
>
> The WHO Traditional Medicine (TM) Strategy 2014–2023 was developed in response to the World Health Assembly resolution on traditional medicine (WHA62.13) (1) (WHO, 2009). The goals of the strategy are to support Member States in:
>
> • harnessing the potential contribution of TM to health, wellness and people centred health care.
> • promoting the safe and effective use of TM by regulating, researching and integrating TM products, practitioners and practice into health systems, where appropriate.
>
> The strategy aims to support Member States in developing proactive policies and implementing action plans that will strengthen the role TM plays in keeping populations healthy. It seeks to build upon the WHO Traditional Medicine Strategy 2002–2005, which reviewed the status of TM globally and in Member States, and set out four key objectives
>
> • policy—integrate TM within national health care systems, where feasible, by developing and implementing national TM policies and programmes.

- safety, efficacy and quality—promote the safety, efficacy and quality of TM by expanding the knowledge base, and providing guidance on regulatory and quality assurance standards.
- access—increase the availability and affordability of TM, with an emphasis on access for poor populations.
- rational use—promote therapeutically sound use of appropriate TM by practitioners and consumers.

United Kingdom, a Case Study: Coordinating Traditional and Complementary Medicine (T&CM) with Western Health Care

WHO (2019, pp. 144–145):

National Policy on T&CM (Traditional and Complementary Medicine)
United Kingdom of Great Britain and Northern Ireland National policy on T&CM In the United Kingdom, the T&CM policy is integrated into the national health policy. There is regulation of OTC herbal medicines under the Traditional Herbal Medicines Regulation (THMR) scheme (Gov.uk, 2021), but there is limited regulation of herbal practitioners or the herbal remedies that they supply to patients following a one-to-one consultation.

The Medicines and Healthcare Products Regulatory Agency and the Department of Health in England have several teams to develop policy on the safe use and practice of T&CM. The Professional Standards section under the Department of Health, in Leeds, is responsible for the professional regulation of practitioners. The Public Health Strategy and Social Marketing section, under the Department of Health, in London, is responsible for policy on CM.

In the United Kingdom, the voluntary sector plays an important facilitating role, and for T&CM this is done by the Prince of Wales Foundation for Integrated Health. The Department of Health has a programme to develop research expertise in T&CM and to strengthen the evidence base. It also commissions periodic surveys of the use of T&CM in the United Kingdom.
Regulatory status of herbal medicines

There are three regulatory routes for herbal medicines in the United Kingdom: unlicensed herbal remedies [covered by s. 12 of the Medicines Act 1968 (legislation.go.uk, 2022)], registered herbal remedies and licensed herbal medicines. The licensed herbal medicines are licensed in the same way as conventional pharmaceuticals; the s. 12 provisions are exclusive to herbal medicines; and the THMR scheme is partly the same as that for conventional pharmaceuticals, but the requirement for efficacy is replaced by proof of traditional use.

Herbal medicines are categorized as prescription medicines, non-prescription medicines and an exclusive regulatory category. They are sold with medical claims. Herbal products not classified as medicines fall within a range of other categories (e.g. foods, food supplements and cosmetics).

The British pharmacopoeia[18] and the European pharmacopoeia are used and are legally binding. The British herbal pharmacopoeia is also used but is not legally binding. Monographs from the British pharmacopoeia (85 British monographs, 244 European monographs) and the European pharmacopoeia (248 monographs) are used and are legally binding. Monographs from the British herbal pharmacopoeia (169 monographs) are not legally binding.

Directive 2003/94/EC (EUR-Lex, 2022) covers GMP for herbal medicines, and the regulations that apply for conventional pharmaceuticals also apply for herbal medicines. Compliance mechanisms include periodic inspections by authorities at the manufacturing plants, and the requirement for manufacturers to assign a person to the role of ensuring compliance. Safety requirements are the same as those for conventional pharmaceuticals.

There are 46 traditional herbal registrations, as of 2012. In addition, there are several hundred herbal medicines with a market authorization. These products are currently being reviewed to assess whether some would more appropriately come within the traditional category. Herbal medicines

---

[18] Medicines & Healthcare products Regulatory Agency (2022) states that:

The BP (British pharmacopoeia) provides the only comprehensive collection of authoritative official standards for UK pharmaceutical substances and medicinal products.

And that monographs provide:
mandatory standards for herbal drugs, herbal drug products and herbal medicinal products, materials for use in the manufacture of homoeopathic preparations

.

are sold in pharmacies and other outlets as non-prescription medicines, self-medication or OTC medicines, and in special outlets.

Practices, providers, education and health insurance

T&CM practices of acupuncture, ayurvedic medicine, chiropractic, herbal medicines, homeopathy, naturopathy, osteopathy, traditional Chinese medicine and Unani medicine are used by the population in the United Kingdom. An estimated 20–39% of the population uses herbal medicines. T&CM providers practise in public and private clinics and hospitals. The regulation of T&CM providers is handled by the Department of Health, but there are two groups that are statutorily regulated (chiropractors and osteopaths). Data on education of T&CM providers and information on coverage of private health insurance are not readily available.

Based on the information shared by the Medicines and Healthcare Products Regulatory Agency (Medicines & Healthcare products Regulatory Agency, 2022), as at 2012, there are an estimated 12,900 acupuncture providers, 3,200 herbal medicine providers and 2,800 traditional Chinese medicine providers in the United Kingdom.

An example of Community Coordination of Traditional Herbal and Complementary Medicine in African Diaspora communities in Greater Manchester.

In view of the UK's National Policy on Traditional & Complementary Medicines (T&CM), a local grassroots training and research institute called MEaP Academy Community Training & Research Institute (MaCTRI) is looking at how it can combine a traditional approach to holistic healthcare with statutory providers within Greater Manchester's Integrated Care System (GMCVO, 2022). Here is what they say on their webpage about their initiative (MaCTRI, 2022):

We are keen to follow the practices set out by the WHO 2014–2023 strategy and the UK's participation in T&CM regulation by setting up a community laboratory and developing an introductory course for herbal practitioners. We are also keen to screen and test the efficacy of herbs native to Nigeria (used by the large Nigerian community in Manchester), which has 4,614 plant species.

We are envisaging a 3-phase proposal

Phase 1—Between May to June 2022, we worked with Masters students in Dietetics from Manchester Metropolitan University to look into public health issues and the use of plant-based preparations either as food, prevention of disease or as treatment. Our survey indicated that over 60% of the respondents (n = 125) indicated that they used of plant preparations for disease prevention or as treatment.

Phase 2—To scale up on phase 1 with NIHR (National Institute for Health and Care Research) funding leading to the establishment of a phytochemical screening laboratory. We will also host Masters students in Pharmacognosy visiting our phytochemical screening laboratory with samples from Department of Pharmacognosy, University of Ibadan in Nigeria in search of bioactive constituents as sources of disease prevention or treatment.

Phase 3—To start delivering courses relating to herbal medicines, phytochemical constituents of plants, medicinal plants and nutraceuticals.

The important points from above are that MaCTRI's research will be directly addressing two of the WHO priorities, namely; "safety, efficacy and quality" and "rational use" in addition to the "regulatory priority" and "education" from the UK's national policy.[19] Led by pharmacognosy-specialist, Dr Esther Olupide, Co-Director of Research at MaCTRI, the research is keen to screen traditional herbal products that are already in use in local majority-Nigerian church communities, with a view to screening the phytochemical purity of the products and conducting trials to evaluate their efficacy. The initiative also seeks to add these products to the British herbal pharmacopoeia after successful trials and written monographs.

---

[19] It is important to note that this work also sits under UN Sustainable Development Goal (SDG) 3, which is all about Health and Well-Being. Also see Clennon (2017) for a UN-commissioned reporting framework for community organisations to be able to use SDG metrics to describe their outputs, allowing for granular analysis of national big data. Especially relevant for the United Nations' International Decade for People of African Descent (IDPAD) 2015–2024 See: https://www.ohchr.org/en/racism/international-decade-african-descent

The Central Role of the Church in African Diaspora Communities

Dr Esther Olupide is also a Pastor at The New Covenant Church in Levenshulme, which is a majority-African (Nigerian) Pentecostal church. This and another Greater Manchester (GM) Pentecostal church were where the participants for the MaCTRI survey were sourced. Dr Oludipe's church also holds CHIPs nights every Thursday, which is a healthy eating initiative and they also run a healing-prayer session[20] once a month. We can see that with the New Covenant Church's healthy eating and healing-prayer initiatives alongside MaCTRI's research into T&CM, there are the definite makings of a holistic system of health prevention that is community-based and culturally sensitive to the health beliefs and needs of its African Diaspora health seekers. The New Covenant Church is also part of a GM-wide network of majority-Black Pentecostal churches called the Upper Room Ministers Forum. The significance of this is that the holistic health initiatives being trialled at the New Covenant Church can be rolled out across the Upper Room Ministers Forum GM network.

In addition to the centrality of the Church in this grassroots initiative between MaCTRI and The New Covenant Church, there is also the exciting prospect of referring community members to an emerging Afrocentric version of Systemic Constellations Practice (SCP) that is being developed by Stuart Taylor, who is a Systems Constellations Practitioner and a MEaP Academy Scholar at MaCTRI[21] (Taylor, forthcoming). SCP comprises a "knowing field"[22] where in a safe and therapeutic space (creating a 'knowing field'), unrelated people to the client are asked to act out family roles and dynamics that are of concern to the

---

[20] See note 7 for literature about the healing power of prayer.

[21] See Stuart Taylor's MaCTRI research page, here: https://critracemmu.wordpress.com/stuart-taylor/

[22] See Clennon (2019) for a personal account of the "knowing field" whose structures deeply resonate with the metaphysical concepts of Sasa and Zamani, discussed previously. Also, important to note that SCP is profoundly influenced by Zulu spirituality, see Taylor (forthcoming).

client. This is a form of expressive therapy[23] and its intention is to assist the client in working through an issue or to gain a better perspective into a conflict.

Conclusion

It is clear to us that the African Model of health, where well-being is broken down into its physical, mental, spiritual and social components, is alive and kicking in our grassroots African Diaspora communities. The grassroots services that comprise this notion of well-being are already being delivered but are mostly under the radar of the wider stakeholders in community and Public Health in Greater Manchester, which means that they are underdeveloped in terms of wider investment.[24] There is huge potential for structured and coordinated partnerships to be brokered between community groups, Churches and wider health stakeholders in Greater Manchester, especially within the context of its Integrated Care System. We can only now hope that the African Diaspora community groups in Greater Manchester will not be left behind in these developments under the mantra of the "hard to reach" because of the effects of whiteness discussed throughout this volume. We also hope that these communities will be able to apply for funding or be commissioned to co-construct ambitious and culturally sensitive health prevention action plans with local statutory providers.[25]

In the next chapter, we will take a wider look at Public Health as it pertains to African Diaspora health seekers. We will examine health policies, their outcomes and the grassroots advocacy work that is being

---

[23] See Clennon (2013) for an example of music being used as an expressive therapy in a mental health context.

[24] See Clennon (2022b) for a report about African Diaspora youth and play provision in Greater Manchester that makes a similar point about underinvestment in African Diaspora communities. However, some important work between the GM Health and Social Care Partnership and Faith Communities has been done but as yet, major investment has not been forthcoming (see MaCTRI, 2017a, b, c, d).

[25] See Lent's et al. (2022, p. para 1) Community-Powered NHS report for a model of "a healthcare system focused as much on preventing illness as treating it. Working collaboratively with communities as equal partners in the design and delivery of healthcare".

undertaken to address the lack of representation at decision-making levels in Public Health in Greater Manchester.

Works Cited

Abu, H. O., Lapane, K. L., Waring, M. E., Ulbricht, C. M., Devereaux, R. S., McManus, D. D., et al. (2019). Religious Practices and Long-Term Survival After Hospital Discharge for an Acute Coronary Syndrome. *PLoS One.* https://doi.org/10.1371/journal.pone.0223442

Akbari, S., Pazokian, M., Farahani, A. S., Nasiri, M., & Rajab, A. (2020). Investigating the Effect of Spiritual Care on the Hope of Diabetic Patients Referred to the Iranian Diabetes Association: A Clinical Trial. *Archives of Pharmacy Practice, 11*(4).

Asante, M. K., & Mazama, A. (Eds.). (2009). *Encyclopedia of African Religion.* Sage.

Billingsley, A. (1999). *Mighty Like a River: The Black Church and Social Reform.* Oxford University Press.

Brown, C. G. (2012). *Testing Prayer.* Harvard University Press.

Burrell, R.-R. (2019). *The Black Majority Church: Exploring the Impact of Faith and a Faith Community on Mental Health and Well-Being.* Middlesex University/Metanoia [Thesis].

Carney, J. A. (2003). African Traditional Plant Knowledge in the Circum-Caribbean Region. *Journal of Ethnobiology, 23*(2), 167–185.

Carter, J. H. (2002). Religion/Spirituality in African American Culture: An Essential Aspect of Psychiatric Care. *Journal of the National Medical Association, 94*(5), 371–375.

Casarez, R. L., & Miles, S. M. (2008). Spirituality: A Cultural Strength for African American Mothers with HIV. *Clinical Nursing Research, 17*(2), 118–132.

Clennon, O. D. (2013). Two Case Examples Using Participatory Music as a Therapy Metaphor in a Community Mental Health Setting in the United Kingdom. *International Journal of Community Music, 6*(1), 33–43.

Clennon, O. D. (2016a). The Black Face of Eurocentrism: Uncovering Globalisation. In O. D. Clennon (Ed.), *International Perspectives of Multiculturalism: The Ethical Challenges* (pp. 91–128). Nova Science.

Clennon, O. D. (2016b). The Ethical Implications of Ideological and Political Multiculturalism in the UK. In O. Clennon (Ed.), *International Perspectives of Multiculturalism: The Ethical Challenges* (pp. 25–69). Nova Science.

Clennon, O. D. (2017, October 30). *SDG Implementation: UK Community Reporting Matrix.* Retrieved from United Nations: Regional Meeting for Europe, Central Asia and North America on the International Decade for People of African Descent: https://www.ohchr.org/en/events/events/2017/regional-meeting-europe-central-asia-and-north-america-international-decade

Clennon, O. D. (2018). *Black Scholarly Activism Between the Academy and Grassroots: A Bridge for Identities and Social Justice.* Palgrave Macmillan.

Clennon, O. D. (2019, September 23). *Systemic Constellations: Creating Our 'Knowing Fields' by Ornette D Clennon.* Retrieved from The Ubele Initiative: https://www.ubele.org/news-and-blog/systemic-constellations-creating-our-knowing-fields-by-ornette-d-clennon

Clennon, O. D. (2022a, June 30). *Visiting an Indigenous Medical Centre.* Retrieved from MaCTRI: https://critracemmu.wordpress.com/visiting-an-indigenous-medical-centre/

Clennon, O. D. (2022b, April 26). *Young Manchester Research: Tackling Racial Injustice.* Retrieved from Young Manchester: https://youngmanchester.org/entry/tackling-racial-injustice

De Sousa Santos, B. (2010). *Epistemologias del sur.* Siglo XXI.

Diessner, S., & Lisi, G. (2020). Masters of the 'Masters of the Universe'? Monetary, Fiscal and Financial Dominance in the Eurozone. *Socio-Economic Review, 18*(2), 315–335.

Dussel, E. (2000). Europe, Modernity, and Eurocentrism. *Nepantla, 1*(3), 465–478.

Dzobo, N. K. (1992). African Symbols and Proverbs as Sources of Knowledge. In K. Wiredu & K. Gyekye (Eds.), *Person and Community: Ghanaian Philosophical Studies I* (Vol. 1, pp. 85–98). Washington.

Emeagwali, G. (2014). Intersections Between Africa's Indigenous Knowledge Systems and History. In G. Emeagwali & G. Sefa Dei (Eds.), *African Indigenous Knowledge and the Disciplines* (pp. 1–19). Sense Publishers.

Erwin, J., & Peters, B. (1999). Treatment Issues for HIV+ Africans in London. *Social Science and Medicine, 49*(11), 1519–1528.

EUR-Lex. (2022, July 8). *Commission Directive 2003/94/EC of 8 October 2003 Laying Down the Principles and Guidelines of Good Manufacturing Practice in Respect of Medicinal Products for Human Use and Investigational Medicinal*

Products for Human Use. Retrieved from EUR-Lex: https://eur-lex.europa.eu/legal-content/EN/TXT/?uri=celex%3A32003L0094

Friedrich-Killinger, S. (2020). Centrality of Religiosity as a Resource for Therapy Outcome? *Religions, 11*(4), 155. https://doi.org/10.3390/rel11040155

Gaiman, N. (2004). *American Gods*. HarperTorch.

George, M. (2012). Health Beliefs, Treatment Preferences and Complementary and Alternative Medicine for Asthma, Smoking and Lung Cancer Self-Management in Diverse Black Communities. *Patient Education and Counseling, 89*(3), 489–500.

GMCVO. (2022, July 11). *Integrated Care Systems*. Retrieved from GMCVO: https://www.gmcvo.org.uk/HSCEngage/IntegratedCareSystems

Gov.uk. (2021, January 5). *Apply for a Traditional Herbal Registration (THR)*. Retrieved from GOV.UK: https://www.gov.uk/guidance/apply-for-a-traditional-herbal-registration-thr

Gross, T. T., Story, C. R., Harvey, I. S., Allsopp, M., & Whitt-Glover, M. (2018). "As a Community, We Need to Be More Health Conscious": Pastors' Perceptions on the Health Status of the Black Church and African-American Communities. *Journal of Racial Ethnic Health Disparities, 5*(3), 570–579.

Gyekye, K. (1995). *An Essay on African Philosophical Thought: The Akan Conceptual Scheme*. Temple University Press.

Harmon, B. E., Strayhorn, S., Webb, B. L., & Hébert, J. R. (2018). Leading God's People: Perceptions of Influence Among African American Pastors. *Journal of Religion and Health, 57*, 1509–1523.

Heward-Mills, N., Atuhaire, C., Spoors, C., Pemunta, N. V., Priebe, G., & Cumber, S. N. (2018). The Role of Faith Leaders in Influencing Health Behaviour: A Qualitative Exploration on the Views of Black African Christians in Leeds, United Kingdom. *Pan African Medical Journal, 30*(199) https://www.panafrican-med-journal.com/content/article/30/199/full

Higginbottom, G. M., & Mathers, N. (2006). The Use of Herbal Remedies to Promote General Wellbeing by Individuals of African-Caribbean Origin in England. *Diversity and Equality in Health and Care, 3*(2), 99–110.

Johnson, K. A. (2018). Prayer: A Helpful Aid in Recovery from Depression. *Journal of Religion and Health, 57*, 2290–2300.

legislation.go.uk. (2022, July 8). *Medicines Act 1968*. Retrieved from legislation.gov.uk: https://www.legislation.gov.uk/ukpga/1968/67/section/12.

Lent, A., Pollard, G., & Studdert, J. (2022, July 12). *A Community-Powered NHS*. Retrieved from New Local: https://www.newlocal.org.uk/publications/community-powered-nhs/

Levin, J. (2009). How Faith Heals: A Theoretical Model. *Explore, 5*(2), 77–96. Available at https://www.sciencedirect.com/science/article/abs/pii/S15508 30708003844

Mackenzie, E. R., Taylor, L., Bloom, B. S., Hufford, D. J., & Johnson, J. C. (2003). Ethnic Minority Use of Complementary and Alternative Medicine (Cam): A National Probability Survey of Cam Utilizers. *Alternative Therapies, 9*(4), 50–56.

MaCTRI. (2017a). *CAHN GM Greater Manchester Health and Social Care Partnership.* Retrieved from MaCTRI: https://critracemmu.wordpress.com/ cahn-gm-greater-manchester-combined-authority-partnership/?frame-nonce=3cb2aeb89e

MaCTRI. (2017b, April 4). *CAHN GM Public Consultations.* Retrieved from MaCTRI: https://critracemmu.wordpress.com/cahn-gm-public-consul tations/?frame-nonce=3cb2aeb89e

MaCTRI. (2017c). *Greater Manchester Health and Social Care Partnership (GMHSCP) Faith Group and Community Services Interim Audit.* Retrieved from MaCTRI: https://critracemmu.wordpress.com/greater-manchester-combined-authority-faith-group-and-community-services-audit/

MaCTRI. (2017d, August 22). *Supporting Sustained Development in BAME Communities: Caribbean and African Faith and Community Leaders Meet Greater Manchester Devolution Leaders, Transformation Community Resource Centre.* Retrieved from MaCTRI: https://critracemmu.wordpress. com/2017/08/09/supporting-sustained-development-in-bame-communi ties-caribbean-and-african-faith-and-community-leaders-meet-greater-manchester-devolution-leaders-command-prayer-centre-22-8-17/

MaCTRI. (2022, July 11). *Research into the Use of Traditional and Complimentary Medicines (TC&M) in the Community.* Retrieved from MaCTRI : https:// critracemmu.wordpress.com/research-into-the-use-of-traditional-and-complimentary-medicines-tcm-in-the-community/

Maier-Lorentz, M. M. (2004). The Importance of Prayer for Mind/Body Healing. *Nursing Forum, 33*(9), 23–32.

Mbiti, J. S. (1970). *African Religions and Philosophy.* Anchor Books.

McGee, S. (2010). *Chasing Goldman Sachs.* Crown Publishing.

Medicines & Healthcare products Regulatory Agency. (2022, July 8). *What Is BP.* Retrieved from The British Pharmacopoeia: https://www.pharmaco-poeia.com/what-is-the-bp

Miranda, T. P., Caldeira, S., de Oliveira, H. F., Iunes, D. H., Nogueira, D. A., de Cássia Lopes Chaves, E., & de Carvalho, E. (2020). Intercessory Prayer on

Spiritual Distress, Spiritual Coping, Anxiety, Depression and Salivary Amylase in Breast Cancer Patients During Radiotherapy: Randomized Clinical Trial. *Journal of Religion and Health, 59*, 365–380.

Newitt, M. (2022). The Clinical Effectiveness of Prayer as an Intervention. *Modern Believing, 63*(3), 259–269.

Nguyen, A. W., Taylor, J. R., Chatters, L. M., & Hope, M. O. (2019). Church Support Networks of African Americans: The Impact of Gender and Religious Involvement. *Journal of Community Psychology, 45*(7), 1043–1063.

Nora, P. (1996). General Introduction: Between Memory and History. In L. D. Krtizmann (Ed.), *Realms of Memory: Rethinking the French Past, Vol. 1: Conflict and Divisions* (A. Goldhammer, Trans., pp. 1–20). Columbia University Press.

Nunn, A., Cornwall, A., Chute, N., Sanders, J., Thomas, G., James, G., et al. (2012, May 16). *Keeping the Faith: African American Faith Leaders' Perspectives and Recommendations for Reducing Racial Disparities in HIV/AIDS Infection.* Retrieved from PLoS One: https://journals.plos.org/plosone/article?id= 10.1371/journal.pone.0036172

Omodara, D., Gibson, L., & Bowpitt, G. (2021). Exploring the Impact of Cultural Beliefs in the Self-Management of Type 2 Diabetes Among Black sub-Saharan Africans in the UK – A Qualitative Study Informed by the PEN-3 Cultural Model. *Ethnicity and Health*, 1–19.

Perdue, B., Johnson, D., Singley, D., & Jackson, C. (2006). Assessing Spirituality in Mentally ill African Americans. *ABNF (Association of Black Nursing Faculty in Higher Education) Journal, 17*(2), 78–81.

Romez, C., Freedman, K., Zaritzky, D., & Brown, J. W. (2021). Case Report of Instantaneous Resolution of Juvenile Macular Degeneration Blindness After Proximal Intercessory Prayer. *Explore, 17*(1), 79–83.

Scott, G. (2010). Traditional Medical Practice in Africa. In S. B. Kayne (Ed.), *Traditional Medicine* (pp. 82–118). Pharmaceutical Press.

Sefa Dei, G. (2014). Indigenizing the Curriculum: The Case of the African University. In G. Emeagwali & G. Sefa Dei (Eds.), *African Indigenous Knowledge and the Disciplines* (pp. 165–180). Sense Publishers.

Sogolo, G. S. (2003). Metaphysical Thinking in Africa: The Concept of Cause in African Thought. In P. H. Coetzee & A. P. Roux (Eds.), *The African Philosophy Reader* (pp. 228–237). Routledge.

Sutherland, P., Moodley, R., & Chevannes, B. (2014). *Caribbean Healing Traditions: Implications for Health and Mental Health*. Routledge.

Taylor, S. (forthcoming). Ancient African Futures: Honouring Our Ancestors a Decolonial Poetics of Restorative Systemic Justice. In O. D. Clennon (Ed.), [book series] *Palgrave Studies in Decolonisation and Grassroots Black Organic Intellectualism*. Palgrave Macmillan.

van Andel, T., Mitchell, S., Volpato, G., Vandebroek, I., Swier, J., Ruysschaert, S., et al. (2012). In Search of the Perfect Aphrodisiac: Parallel Use of Bitter Tonics in West Africa and the Caribbean. *Journal of Ethnopharmacology, 143*(3), 840–850.

Waghid, Y., & Smeyers, P. (2012). Reconsidering Ubuntu: On the Educational Potential of a Particular Ethic of Care. *Educational Philosophy and Theory, 44*(S2), 6–20.

WHO. (2009, May 18–22). *Sixty-Second World Health Assembly.* Retrieved from World Health Organization: https://apps.who.int/gb/ebwha/pdf_files/WHA62-REC1/WHA62_REC1-en.pdf.

WHO. (2013). *WHO Traditional Medicine Strategy: 2014–2023.* Retrieved from World Health Organisation: https://apps.who.int/iris/handle/10665/92455?search-result=true&query=WHO+global+report+on+traditional+and+complementary+medicine+2022+africa&scope=%2F&rpp=10&sort_by=score&order=desc&page=3

WHO. (2019). *WHO Global Report on Traditional and Complementary Medicine 2019.* World Health Organization. Available at https://www.who.int/news/item/20-05-2019-the-who-global-report-on-traditional-and-complementary-medicine-2019-is-released

Williams, L. F., & Cousin, L. (2021). "A Charge to Keep I Have": Black Pastors' Perceptions of Their Influence on Health Behaviors and Outcomes in Their Churches and Communities. *Journal of Religion and Health, 60*, 1069–1082.

5

Where Do We Go from Here? Decolonised Health Advocacy

Abstract In this chapter, we will present an in-depth case study of an African Diaspora-led health advocacy organisation in Greater Manchester, called Caribbean & African Health Network (CAHN). We will explore how in advocating for better health outcomes by dialoguing with regional and national stakeholders within the health market, they are assuming the role of "grassroots Black organic intellectual" (Gordon, Black Intellectual Tradition. Retrieved from Genius: https://genius.com/Lewis-gordon-black-intellectual-tradition-annotated, 2009) in their local grassroots communities and beyond. The case study will present how they are able to successfully translate their decolonial scholarship around health into health policy and health advocacy for African Diaspora communities in the UK, as they build regional and national partnerships with systems leaders.

Keywords Grassroots Black organic intellectual • Health advocacy • African Diaspora health • Decolonial praxis

F. Bruce, O. D. Clennon, *Decolonising Public Health through Praxis*,
https://doi.org/10.1007/978-3-031-18405-5_5

Introduction

In the previous chapter, we outlined a community initiative led by MEaP Academy Community Training & Research Institute (MaCTRI) that was dedicated to re-discovering "traditional heritage knowledges" around traditional and complementary medicines (T&CM). We outlined how MaCTRI is building its decolonial praxis with its Church partnerships that allows it to simultaneously explore decoloniality and decolonisation in the area of traditional community health practices. In this chapter, we will primarily look at another Manchester-based organisation called Caribbean & African Health Network (CAHN). CAHN grew out of a decolonial doctoral research project into the hidden factors behind health disparities in African Diaspora communities. Since its inception, CAHN has become Greater Manchester's leading African Diaspora community organisation advocating for better Black health investment at both grassroots and policy levels with the Greater Manchester Combined Authority (GMCA). This is significant because in 2016, health was devolved to GMCA from Westminster with a £6 billon health and social care budget (Gov.uk, 2016). This means that the spending priorities of this budget are now decided by Greater Manchester Health and Social Care Partnership (GMHSCP) rather than by the Department of Health in Westminster. So, there are even fewer excuses for funding "cold spots" when it comes to tackling health disparities in Greater Manchester's African Diaspora communities and ethnic minority communities more widely.

Caribbean & African Health Network (CAHN): A Case Study

Our community conversations have revealed a range of contemporary barriers and gaps in access to the health market that have their roots in the historical patterns of behaviour that is, whiteness. This has required a combination of post and decolonial scholarship, health advocacy and political activism in order to mount a sustained community campaign for structural change within the health sector. This shift to address poor health has resulted in the development of the Caribbean & African Health Network (CAHN), whose aim is to decolonise universal Eurocentric health-knowledges through our collective community grass-roots advocacy organisations. The purpose is to end health disparities in a generation and to do this in a way that dismantles the ways in which Black health is poorly managed. As an organisation, the rich intergenerational intelligence gathered from across Black communities of identity highlights the way in which Black people's view of health and health-seeking are experienced in starkly different ways (to white people) and how these experiences require a more diverse response that actually meets their needs.

A rich research base including contributions from CAHN's partners and community members since the establishment of CAHN, underpins the work to decolonise public health and improve health outcomes (CAHN, 2022a). As discussed throughout this volume, we can see that structural systems, policies, practices and processes do not provide equity for black people in health prevention and improvement. CAHN works with systems to deconstruct these barriers. CAHN has worked to create a platform or engine room with policy makers, health professionals, researchers and patients with lived experiences to change the experience of cardiovascular disease in the Black community (CAHN, 2022a). The essence of this work is to develop tested ways that work to engage our community but one that is resourced and sustained over the Integrated Care System[1] footprints.

In tandem with this work, is the importance of building trust with research institutions because the evidence-base about what works for our communities is essential for appropriate care and treatment. CAHN has found that there is limited engagement with agencies in healthcare including research institutions for a number of reasons. Lessons from the past have resulted in a lack of trust[2] and CAHN witnessed this lack of trust during the height of the pandemic where over 72 percent of Black people were hesitant to take the COVID-19 vaccine (Geddes, 2021).

---

[1] See Chap. 4.
[2] See Chaps. 2, 3 and 4.

The historical patterns of whiteness and its epigenetic changes[3] provide us with an understanding of how the historical origins of whiteness have resulted in higher rates of mortality and morbidity for Black people. As discussed in Chap. 3, genetics and biological models of health have often been used to explain the root causes of poor health within Black communities. However, the stressors of racism and its epigenetic effects are better able to explain why Black people are more at risk of higher rates of morbidity and mortality across many health conditions, including COVID-19. Recent medical reactions to COVID-19 have tried to attribute the disproportionately high rate of COVID-19 deaths from Black communities on genes that leave Black people more vulnerable to contracting the virus and dying.[4] However, studies have argued the epigenetic case for the interaction between structural discrimination and negative health outcomes (e.g. Graff, 2014; Shackel, 2018),[5] increasing the call to see race as a social determinant of health. There have also been epigenetic studies that have looked at the effect of stress and how it is transmitted from the mother to the foetus in the prenatal period (e.g. Weaver, 2007). However, other studies have gone beyond that to identify the long term and intergenerational trauma of stress, resulting from slavery (e.g. Jackson et al., 2014; DeGruy Leary, 2005).

Using the knowledge of whiteness and its epigenetic changes, CAHN as a grassroots upstream advocacy organisation is built on the legacy of community action that seeks to empower, enable and equip faith and community organisations to deliver and shape health and well-being services. It recognises how knowledge that has been traditionally produced by western thinkers devalues Black voices whilst promoting the voices of the powerful (Elabor-Idemudia, 2011). The lack of Black voices has made it difficult to address issues affecting Black people because public health knowledge is constructed and shaped through the eyes of a colonial education system and its historical patterns of whiteness (Verweijen & Van Bockhaven, 2020).[6] So, CAHN was developed from a movement that

---

[3] See Chaps. 2 and 3.
[4] See Chap. 3.
[5] See Chap. 3 for more details.
[6] See Chap. 3.

heard these missing voices and a movement that uncovered the hidden practices of whiteness that needed to be uncovered and addressed in order to bring about justice and fairness. Throughout the evolution of the community conversations that founded CAHN, racism was clearly recognised and acknowledged as a key factor that was significantly relevant to public health. However, the field of healthcare and research in the production of knowledge has largely ignored how relevant race is when addressing health disparities in the UK.

CAHN as an Infrastructure Organisation

As discussed in Chap. 3, some of the negative legacies of slavery and colonialism, such as self-hate, anti-African sentiments and a lack of pride in being Black have been internalised in our communities (DeGruy Leary, 2005). This internalised behaviour can be passed down intergenerationally. DeGruy Leary (2005) argues that Black people should view their behaviours and attitudes through the colonial lens of history to understand the impact and influence of slavery and colonialism on their attitudes today. CAHN specifically facilitates this process of consciousness-raising (i.e. Paulo Freire's "conscientisation", Freire, 1973 or more specifically decolonial thinking; see Mignolo & Escobar, 2010; Mignolo, 2000, 2002).

Our community partners have been clear that although there are strong internal (community) foundational relationships especially through the church and religion,[7] there are also some community challenges that result in the fragmentation and breakdown of community relations and bonding. When unpacking the historical basis for this fragmentation, we find that community rivalry and anti-African sentiments (the remnants of colonialism) explain the basis for some of this disharmony resulting in the "crabs in the barrel syndrome" (Miller, 2019). Our community members often tell us that commissioners use this fragmentation and rivalry as a reason not to fund community organisations adequately. So, CAHN believes that future work is most definitely needed to

---

[7] See Chap. 4.

explore how funding can be used to encourage intra-community coop-eration in the form of soliciting consortium bids for tender.[8]

In response to this fragmentation, the CAHN network brings together Caribbean and African-led organisations to work together so that they can effectively engage statutory providers to respond to their challenging health disparities. In our conversations, community members tell us that this work requires joined-up working with Black-led communities and efficient coordination to enable it to be efficient and effective. Through continued community consultation and engagement CAHN has to date attracted over 5000 community organisations (including Black majority churches) and individuals that want to be part of this movement that provides appropriate custom-made services for our Caribbean and African Communities (CAHN, 2022b).

Due to the lack of value placed in Black epistemological knowledge, gaps in mainstream provision have stubbornly persisted and have led many communities to set up their own organisations to address the needs of Black people. Historically, Black-led organisations were largely set up in the 1950s when many people from the Caribbean and later on from the African Continent were invited to fill jobs after World War II (Olwig, 2017). These organisations have notoriously been underfunded by gov-ernment agencies, as previously discussed, leaving Black people to con-tinue to be challenged with unmet health needs. Our community partners speak about how first and foremost, these organisations provide cultur-ally appropriate information to help navigate Black people through an unequal system in the UK. Our community members also complain that even though their services are often cited as valuable to the community, their value is not reflected in the overall decisions that agencies make to fund their work or even address their health needs. This is even the case when Black-led organisations provide evidence of impact with accompa-nying research to prove that they are best placed to meet the needs of Black people (Memon et al., 2016). As community partners state, they lack sufficient investment by agencies and more often than not, lose out to larger national VCSE sector organisations that are not representative

---

[8] See Chap. 4 and Clennon (2022) for a report into the need for consortium bidding from African Diaspora community service providers.

of their community (Clennon, 2022). Our community partners strongly suggest that there appears to be a bias in decision-making (Clennon, 2022). We have found that decision-making that positively impacts health is generally only afforded to white people (especially from wealthier socio-economic backgrounds) who tend to be in networks where they share power and privilege that are often denied to Black people.[9] The public health landscape has failed to include race and racism as a social determinant of health, which has had a deleterious effect on policy making for Black health. For example, in 2019, CAHN challenged Sir Michael Marmot by asking him why he thought that race and racism were not determinants of health; he responded that there was not enough evidence (Bruce, 2020). However, Marmot (2020, p. 23) has since included race/ethnicity as part of his determinants of health, which we suspect is as a result of the data coming from early-wave COVID-19 rates of infections:

> Intersections between socioeconomic status, ethnicity and racism intensify inequalities in health for ethnic groups.

CAHN has built stronger relationships within our communities and with other stakeholders to facilitate awareness, to develop culturally specific resources, to facilitate social inclusion, equity and as a result, to improve the life chances of disadvantaged communities. However, CAHN has found that even when representatives of Black organisations are around the decision-making table, their experience and expertise around the health needs of Black communities are often ignored, as it is often the case that they exist as an "othered" individual or a tick box exercise (token).

The emergence of CAHN represents how Black people currently negotiate the health market but also how they can more effectively negotiate the health market in the *future*. The initiative aims to work in partnership with Caribbean and African people to develop the education, awareness and health literacy skills in order to have a better chance to improve the health and well-being of our communities. CAHN currently works collaboratively with commissioners, statutory and voluntary sector

---

[9] See Chap. 2 about whiteness and gatekeeping.

organisations with an emphasis on sustaining health and well-being pro-vision within the Caribbean and African community. The organisation has a focus on facilitating capacity-building in the Caribbean and African voluntary and community sectors in order for them to better able to work in partnerships with wider stakeholders.

CAHN is a trusted voice for Black people in Greater Manchester.[10] For example, in response to a specific community request, CAHN advocated on the communities' behalf to Greater Manchester (GM) Health & Social Care Partners about maternal mortality and actions to address the GM-reflection of national rates that report that Black women in preg-nancy or shortly after delivery are five times more likely to die. Although it took several months to gather the data, due to poor ethnic data collec-tion, it was identified that Greater Manchester's picture of maternal mor-tality (Khan, 2021; Firdous et al., 2020) reflected the MBRRACE-UK's data[11] showing that Black women are indeed five times more likely to die in pregnancy or shortly after delivery (Knight, 2019). Conversations between strategic partners and CAHN then began to determine what needed to be done to improve maternal outcomes.[12] In their quest to respond to their community enquiry, CAHN also challenged a provider organisation in Manchester (NHS Race & Health Observatory, 2022) to look into near misses as they collected narratives from Black women, which highlighted the incidence of sometimes discriminatory and racist practice resulting in long term medical and psychological harms.[13] CAHN and other VCSE partners collaborated with our maternity system to produce standards that have been built on the voices of our Black and Asian women, birthing people and families (NHS England - Northwest, 2022). This has resulted in a Greater Manchester and Eastern Cheshire mandate, which states that each provider needs to work towards ensuring these standards are implemented, monitored and reviewed.

---

[10] See Chap. 4 about community trust building.

[11] "MBRRACE-UK is the collaboration appointed by the Healthcare Quality Improvement Partnership (HQIP) to run the national Maternal, Newborn and Infant clinical Outcome Review Programme (MNI-CORP)" taken from https://www.npeu.ox.ac.uk/mbrrace-uk#:~:text=' MBRRACE%2DUK'%20is%20the,the%20causes%20of%20maternal%20deaths%2C

[12] For Black women (five times more likely to die). Mixed-race women (three times more likely to die) and Asian women (twice as likely to die).

[13] See Chap. 2.

Commentary

Black Beetle Health

At this point it is also worth mentioning the Sheffield-based online grass-roots organisation called Black Beetle Health (2022a), who are a youth-led organisation dedicated to promoting health, well-being and equality to LGBTQ+ Black and People of Colour. Even though they deliver their services primarily online, a substantial number of their service users are based in Greater Manchester.

> The Health Equity and Advocacy Programme (H.E.A.T.) is a cultural safety development tool for individuals engaging with LGBTQ+ Black and People of Colour across Health, Wellbeing and Equality in the UK. This programme was designed to improve understanding, discussion, and decolonisation of theories and practices that continue to feed the appetite of ill health and present a range of health disparities for LGBTQ+ Black and People of Colour (BPoC) in the widest definition of the phrase.
>
> Outcomes captured from the rollout and delivery of the H.E.A.T. Programme pilot clearly demonstrate the impact of funded training initiatives that highlight the specific needs of racially and sexually minoritised individuals and address health inequalities impacting these communities.
>
> Having engaged a range of voices, incorporating the recommendations and comments from participants will inform the programme's direction as well as impact other projects and courses we may develop in future.
>
> (2022b, para 2)

In their H.E.A.T programme, it is particularly interesting to note their focus on the following (Kennedy-Pitt, 2021, p. 5):

Module 3: Decolonising the Colonised
• Understand the term 'colonisation' and its historical role in health inequalities.
• Provide a brief overview of the negative impact of colonisation on health wellbeing and equality for LGBTQ+ BPoC.

- Provide examples of how decolonisation initiatives can be implemented across health, education, business, and society.

Providing online training that explicitly provides the space to discuss what colonisation means in terms of health inequalities and especially within an LGBTQ+ and BPoC context is also a great example of grassroots Black organic intellectualism in practice (Gordon, 2009). Also see below for an outline of their module 7 (Kennedy-Pitt, 2021, p. 7):

- Understand community approaches to health intervention.
- Discuss the importance of community-led work.
- Describe ways in which we can place communities at the centre of our practice.

The above excerpt is particularly significant for the conscious process of building a decolonial health praxis in the community. The importance of grassroots-led health provision for maximum health outcomes for African Diaspora health seekers cannot be overstated.

Conclusion

In this chapter, we have attempted to provide a snapshot of some of the radical work being done in our grassroots African Diaspora communities around health. Throughout this volume, the voices of our community partners have played a central role in the development of a decolonial praxis where decolonial theory is discussed by the community, for the community and applied to the community, by the community. In short, a decolonial praxis for the empowerment and liberation of African Diaspora communities across Greater Manchester.

It is clear that in these times of dwindling resources and a "cost of living crisis" that genuine, fair and radical partnership-building between statutory providers and African Diaspora service providers is needed more than ever for equitable resourcing and investment in these communities. As we have argued throughout this volume, whiteness and its historical patterns of behaviour are ethical and moral issues that underpin inequity of access to health services for African Diaspora health seekers and within this ethical framework, these issues become an urgent question of civil rights!

We hope that this volume sparks and adds to the ongoing debate at grassroots and policy levels about how we are going to action real transformative change, *together* for our communities in this most challenging of times.

Works Cited

Black Beetle Health. (2022a, July 27). *About.* Retrieved from Black Beetle Health: https://www.blackbeetlehealth.co.uk/

Black Beetle Health. (2022b, July 27). *Health Education and Promotion.* Retrieved from Black Beetle Health: https://www.blackbeetlehealth.co.uk/health-education-and-promotion.

Bruce, F. (2020). *Decolonising Health Inequalities: Uncovering the Hidden Factors Behind Biological Models of Caribbean and African Health Outcomes in Greater Manchester.* [PhD thesis] Retrieved from e-space.mmu.ac.uk: https://e-space.mmu.ac.uk/628441/1/FB%20PhD%20final%202021.pdf

CAHN. (2022a, July 18). *Reports.* Retrieved from CAHN: https://www.cahn.org.uk/reports/

CAHN. (2022b, July 27). *Scoping.* Retrieved from CAHN: https://www.cahn.org.uk/research/scoping/

Clennon, O. D. (2022, April 26). *Young Manchester Research: Tackling Racial Injustice.* Retrieved from Young Manchester: https://youngmanchester.org/entry/tackling-racial-injustice.

DeGruy Leary, J. (2005). *Post Traumatic Slave Syndrome: America's Legacy of Enduring Injury and Healing.* Uptone Press.

Elabor-Idemudia, P. (2011). Identity, Representation and Knowledge Production. *Counterpoints, 379*, 142–156.

Firdous, T., Darwin, Z., & Hassan, S. M. (2020). Muslim Women's Experiences of Maternity Services in the UK: Qualitative Systematic Review and Thematic Synthesis. *BMC Pregnancy and Childbirth, 20*(15). https://doi.org/10.1186/s12884-020-2811-8

Freire, P. (1973). *Pedagogy of the Oppressed.* Seabury Press.

Geddes, L. (2021, January 16). *Covid Vaccine: 72% of Black People Unlikely to Have Jab, UK Survey Finds.* Retrieved from The Guardian: https://www.theguardian.com/world/2021/jan/16/covid-vaccine-black-people-unlikely-covid-jab-uk

Gordon, L. (2009). *Black Intellectual Tradition.* Retrieved from Genius: https://genius.com/Lewis-gordon-black-intellectual-tradition-annotated

Gov.uk. (2016, May). *Devolution: A Mayor for Greater Manchester. What Does It Mean?* Retrieved from assets.publishing.service.gov.uk: https://assets.publishing.service.gov.uk/government/uploads/system/uploads/attachment_data/file/608528/Plain_English_Guides_to_Devolution_Greater_Manchester.pdf

Graff, G. (2014). The Intergenerational Trauma of Slavery and Its Aftermath. *The Journal of Psychohistory, 41*(3), 181–197.

Jackson, F. M., Saran, A. R., Ricks, S., Essien, J., Klein, K., Roberts, D., & Worthy, N. (2014). Save 100 Babies (c): Engaging Communities for Just and Equitable Birth Outcomes Through Photovoice and Appreciative Inquiry. *Maternal and Child Health Journal, 18*(9), 1786–1794.

Kennedy-Pitt, H. A. (2021). *H.E.A.T Programme Pilot Support.* Black Beetle Health.

Khan, Z. (2021). Ethnic Health Inequalities in the UK's Maternity Services: A Systematic Literature Review. *British Journal of Midwifery, 29*, 100–107.

Knight, M. (2019). The Findings of the MBRRACE-UK Confidential Enquiry into Maternal Deaths and Morbidity. *Obstetrics, Gynaecology and Reproductive Medicine, 29*(1), 21–23.

Marmot, M. (2020, February). *Health Equity in England: The Marmot Review 10 Years On.* Retrieved from The Health Foundation: https://www.health.org.uk/publications/reports/the-marmot-review-10-years-on

Memon, A., Taylor, K., Mohebati, L. M., Sundin, J., Cooper, M., Scanlon, T., & de Visser, R. (2016). Perceived Barriers to Accessing Mental Health Services Among Black and Minority Ethnic (BME) Communities: A Qualitative Study in Southeast England. *BMJ Open, 16*(6) https://bmjopen.bmj.com/content/6/11/e012337

Mignolo, W. (2000). *Local Histories/Global Designs: Essays on the Coloniality of Power, Subaltern Knowledges and Border Thinking.* Princeton University Press.

Mignolo, W. (2002). The Geopolitics of Knowledge and the Colonial Difference. *South Atlantic Quarterly, 101*(1), 57–96.

Mignolo, W. D., & Escobar, A. (Eds.). (2010). *Globalization and the Decolonial Option.* Routledge.

Miller, C. D. (2019). Exploring the Crabs in the Barrel Syndrome in Organisations. *Journal of Leadership and Organisational Studies, 26*(3), 352–371.

NHS England - Northwest. (2022, July 27). *Maternity Safety Information.* Retrieved from NHS England: https://www.england.nhs.uk/north-west/north-west-services/north-west-maternity-services/maternity-safety-information/

NHS Race & Health Observatory. (2022, 27 July). *Homepage.* Retrieved from NHS Race & Health Observatory: https://www.nhsrho.org/.

Olwig, K. F. (2017). Female Immigration and the Ambivalence of Dirty Care Work: Caribbean Nurses in Imperial Britain. *Ethnography, 19*(1), 44–62.

Shackel, P. A. (2018). Transgenerational Impact of Structural Violence: Epigenetics and the Legacy of Anthracite Coal. *International Journal of Historical Archaeology, 22*(4), 865–882.

Verweijen, J., & Van Bockhaven, V. (2020). Revisiting Colonial Legacies in Knowledge Production on Customary Authority in Central and East Africa. *Journal of Eastern African Studies, 14*(1), 1–23.

Weaver, I. C. (2007). Epigenetic Programming by Maternal Behaviour and Pharmacological Intervention - Nature Versus Nurture: Let's Call the Whole Thing Off. *Epigenetics, 2*(1), 22–28.

Correction to: Decolonising Public Health: What Are the Alternatives?

Correction to:

Chapter 4 in: F. Bruce, O. D. Clennon, *Decolonising Public Health through Praxis*, https://doi.org/10.1007/978-3-031-18405-5_4

Chapter "Decolonising Public Health: What Are the Alternatives?" was previously published with an error "Zumani" and has now been corrected to "Zamani".

The updated version of this chapter can be found at
https://doi.org/10.1007/978-3-031-18405-5_4

C1

Printed in the United States
by Baker & Taylor Publisher Services